U0313679

全国高等院校数字化课程规划教材

供护理、助产及医学相关专业使用

护理英语（听说分册）

English for Nursing (Listening and Speaking)

主　编　罗　渝　刘　琦

副主编　胡晓莉　曾艾玲　穆　艳　吕小君

编　者　（按姓氏汉语拼音排序）

方露燕　金华职业技术学院

胡晓莉　山东医学高等专科学校

李婉瑄　广州卫生职业技术学院

刘　琦　承德护理职业学院

刘　青　泰山护理职业学院

罗　渝　广州卫生职业技术学院

吕小君　承德护理职业学院

穆　艳　铁岭卫生职业学院

谢颖怡　惠州卫生职业技术学院

于　婷　泰山护理职业学院

袁　文　承德护理职业学院

张媛媛　长沙卫生职业学院

曾艾玲　惠州卫生职业技术学院

科学出版社

北　京

内 容 简 介

本教材为了顺应医药卫生事业的发展和行业对人才素质要求的不断提高而编写，旨在提高学生的专业英语口语能力，特别是学生同病患、病患家属或其他医务工作者使用行业英语沟通的口语表达能力。教材编写中，我们围绕章节主题设计多个任务，以口语任务为主，完成工作场景中可能遇到的模拟任务（如采集病史、生命体征测量、交班、用药指导等）；以听力任务为辅，为学生做好语言输入和积累。

本教材可供护理、助产及医学相关专业使用。

图书在版编目（CIP）数据

护理英语（听说分册）＝English for Nursing (Listening and Speaking) / 罗渝，刘琦主编. —北京：科学出版社，2019.9

全国高等院校数字化课程规划教材

ISBN 978-7-03-060308-1

Ⅰ. 护… Ⅱ. ①罗… ②刘… Ⅲ. 护理学－英语－听说教学－高等学校－教材 Ⅳ. R47

中国版本图书馆CIP数据核字（2019）第001085号

责任编辑：张立丽 许 岚／责任校对：王 瑞
责任印制：徐晓晨／封面设计：金舵手世纪

科 学 出 版 社 出版

北京东黄城根北街16号
邮政编码：100717
http://www.sciencep.com

北京盛通商印快线网络科技有限公司 印刷

科学出版社发行 各地新华书店经销

＊

2019年9月第 一 版 开本：787×1092 1/16
2021年7月第三次印刷 印张：14 1/4
字数：335 000

定价：45.00 元

（如有印装质量问题，我社负责调换）

前　言

　　根据《高等职业学校专业教学标准（试行）》和《高职高专教育英语课程教学基本要求（试行）》"以实用为主，以应用为目的"的要求，本教材结合岗位需求分析，旨在提高学生的医护专业英语口语能力，特别是医护人员同病患、病患家属或其他医务工作者使用行业英语沟通的口语表达能力，希望培养出来的学生可以胜任国内普通医院和外资医疗机构的涉外医护工作，甚至能在国际医护专业市场找到一席之地。

　　本教材可供护理、助产及医学相关专业使用。教材编写中，我们围绕章节主题设计多个任务，以听力任务为辅，为学生做好语言输入和积累；以口语任务为主，完成工作场景中可能遇到的模拟任务（如采集病史、生命体征测量、交班、用药指导等）。

　　结合学生的认知水平、职业需求的特点，本教材在内容选材、教学方法、学习方法等方面以"必需、够用、实用"为原则，注重学生积累 input，然后转化成内在的能力，变成 output，不追求过分复杂的句型句式，以专业培养目标为导向，以职业技能的培养为根本，加强与专业实际应用的联系，通过完成职场任务，培养学生解决实际问题及创新的能力。

　　本教材包括 15 个单元，可以安排 1～2 个学期使用。单元基本框架如下。

• Lead-in

　　此部分提供该章节常用句子，激活学生的相关知识，为学习本单元积累必要的 input。

• Tasks

　　每个单元由 9 个任务（tasks）组成，9 个任务以单元主题为统一线索，主题下又分为 3 个分话题，都是医护工作中常见的场景和情境，听说任务活动形式多样，不拘一格。

• More Practice

　　每一章节最后的 More Practice，通过一个相关案例，设计 OET 口语考试练习模板，加强学生 critical thinking 的能力，帮助他们学会解决临床问题。

　　本书在编写过程中得到了所有编者的积极配合，在此表示诚挚的谢意。由于编者水平有限，编写时间仓促，书中难免有疏漏，敬请读者批评指正。

编　者

2019 年 7 月

Contents

Admitting Patients

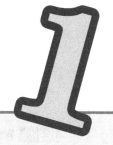

Intended Learning Objectives

On completion of the unit, students should be able to:

1. talk about hospital departments;
2. receive a patient on admission;
3. collect patients' information.

Lead-in

Listen and repeat. 🎧

Listen to the following sentences and repeat them. Pay attention to the pronunciation and intonation.

1. Good morning, Mr. Brown. My name is Cindy. I'll be the nurse looking after you today.
2. Would you mind if I ask you a few questions? / We need some information from you.
3. Can you tell me your full name and date of birth, please?
4. I'd like to know why you're here today.
5. Do you have any allergies to medications?
6. Can you tell me the name of your next of kin?
7. I'd like to know the phone number of your next of kin.
8. What is your job? /Could you tell me your occupation?
9. Do you have any serious illnesses in the past?
10. Please wait a moment. I'll let your doctor know. / I'll inform your doctor.

> **Communication Focus**
> **Self-introduction and greetings are expected before healthcare transactions occur.**
>
> *In pairs, discuss the following questions.*
> 1. What are the main responsibilities of a hospital receptionist?
> 2. If you are a ward nurse, how do you introduce yourself to the patient and make greetings?

Part One Talking About Hospital Departments

Task 1 **Work in pairs.**

Match the following signs to the department names below. Explain what may happen in that hospital setting to your partner.

Example: *In consulting room, …*

a   b   c   d

e   f   g   h

( ) 1. Nurse Station   ( ) 2. Operating Room

( ) 3. Consulting Room   ( ) 4. Pharmacy

( ) 5. Medical Department   ( ) 6. Ward

( ) 7. Surgical Department   ( ) 8. Emergency Room

Task 2 **Pronounce the words.** 🎧

Write down the words according to the phonetic symbols below. And then listen and check.

1. / i'mɜːdʒənsi / _____   2. / ˌpiːdi'ætrɪks / _____

3. / 'sɜːdʒəri / _____   4. / mə'tɜːnəti / _____

5. / ˌdʒeri'ætrɪks / _____   6. / ˌreɪdi'ɒlədʒi / _____

Task 3 **Listen and complete.** 🎧

Listen to the following sentences carefully and fill in the missing words. Then read the sentences with your partner.

1. Pediatric Dept. is where they treat _____.

2. Surgical Dept. is where surgeons carry out _____.

3. Emergency Room is the place where they treat _____.

4. Radiology Dept. is where they _____.

5. Midwives deliver _____ in the Maternity Unit.

6. Specialists in geriatrics treat problems related to the _____.

Part Two Receiving Patient on Admission

Task 4 **Work in pairs.** 🎧

Put the following sentences in the correct order and then listen to the conversation and check your answer.

☐ Sure. Patients usually get up at 7: 00 a. m. Breakfast is at 8: 00 a. m. The ward rounds and treatment start

at 9: 00 a. m. After lunch you could have a nap or rest. Visiting hours are from 3: 00 p. m. to 7: 00 p. m.
Supper is at 6: 00 p. m. Bed time is from 9: 30 p. m. to 10: 00 p. m. And we provide hot water 24 hours.

☐ OK. That's fine.

☐ Of course, it is over there at the corner. And do you need clean pajamas?

☐ Please let us know if you need any help, and smoking is not allowed here.

☐ Thank you. Will you show me where the bathroom is?

☐ Good morning, Mr. Green. My name is Sarah, I'm in charge of this ward. If you need anything, please press this button.

☐ Yes, please. Is it possible for my family to stay here with me?

☐ Good morning, Sarah. Could you tell me the hours here for having meals and visiting?

☐ We don't think it is necessary, since your condition isn't so serious.

Task 5 Work in pairs. 🎧

Put these words in order to make sentences. Discuss the details of one patient which the nurse should take down in admission. Listen and check your answers.

1. Caroline, morning, Good, trouble, to, so, sorry, I'm, you, much.

2. nurse, the, Welcome, in, charge, of, this, Mrs. Johnson, department, I'm, Daisy.

3. mind, check, if, I, Would, you, out, details, of, some, you?

4. would, to, What, you, like, know?

5. your, name, and, date, check, of, I'd, like, to, birth.

6. name, is, Catherine Jonathan, full, My, and, birth, my, the, fifth, of, July, nineteen, fifty, seven, date, is, the, of.

7. bring, your, bedside, Please, me, follow, to, I'll, you.

8. supply, water, hot, the, is, toilet, over, there, We, and.

9. let, us, you, if, any, need, help, Please, know.

10. allowed, not, Smoking, is, here.

Task 6 Role-play. 🎧

Play the role and listen to the sample.

Scenario: in the reception room

Task: Student A plays as a nurse to get information for Student B. And swap the role later.

Useful sentence patterns:

1. I'd like to check your personal details, is that okay?

2. Could you tell me your full name, please?

3. Can you spell that, please?

4. What would you like us to call you?

5. Where are you from?

6. I'm originally from Chicago. But I came here for my studies. I got married, and now I'm looking forward to my first child. I've been here for ten years already.

7. What is your date of birth and what is your job?

8. I also need to ask who your next of kin is to contact in an emergency.

9. My husband, Daniel Miller, is my next of kin. His mobile number is 0677-998-7787.

10. Do you have any allergies?

Part Three Taking Patient History

Task 7 Work in pairs.

A. Read the patient record and answer the questions.

Patient Record	
Surname: Stewart	**First name:** Richard
DOB: 21/2/1982	**Gender:** M̌ F
Occupation: supermarket manager	
Marital status: married	**Next of kin:** Celina, wife
Contact No. : 08277 8392	**Smoking intake:** n/a
Alcohol intake: 20 units per week	**Reason for admission:** dog bite
Medical history: high blood pressure	**Allergy:** n/a
Email: Ric. 0201Woods@hotmail. com	**Address:** 177 Riverdale, Linden Street
GP: Dr. Philip. Central Surgery	

1. What's the patient's name?

2. Is the patient a man or a woman?

3. When is the patient's birthday?

4. What is the patient's job?

5. Who is Dr. Philip?

B. Find words and abbreviations in the patient record with the same meanings.

1. family doctor _____GP_____

2. date of birth _____

3. bad reactions, for example to certain medications _____

4. male/female _____

5. job _____

6. married/single/divorced/widowed _____

7. past illnesses and injuries _____

8. closest relatives _____

9. not applicable _____

Task 8 **Listen and complete.** 🎧

Listen to the audio and complete the chart. And act it out in pairs.

ID Bracelet	
Full name	
DOB	
Hospital No.	
Allergy	
Next of kin	
Contact No.	

Task 9 **Work in pairs.**

Prepare nurse-patient conversation with useful sentences.

A. student A: You are a nurse and student B is a patient. Ask student B questions to complete this Patient Details.

Patient Detail	
Name	
Gender	
DOB	
Country of origin	
Job	
Next of kin	
Relationship to patient	
Allergy	

B. student B: You are a patient, and student A is a nurse. Below is your detailed information. Answer student A's questions using this.

Your name is Marilyn Stuart, female. Your date of birth is 12th July 1979. You are from America and now work as a fashion designer. Edison Stuart is your next of kin and husband. You are allergic to morphine.

Useful sentences

1. Have you got an ID bracelet on?
2. Can I look at your ID bracelet, please?
3. Can you tell me your full name, please?
4. What's your date of birth, please?
5. Do you have any allergies?
6. Can you tell me the name of your next of kin?

More Practice

Role-play.

Read the following case and play the roles of a nurse and a patient based on the case. In the dialogue, you should complete the tasks below the case.

> **Case Study:** Mr. Jim Green is a 59-year-old man who works as a taxi driver. He is a heavy smoker. He was admitted to the hospital with bronchitis. You are asked to obtain personal details from the patient and to respond to the patient's questions about giving up smoking.

Tasks:

1. Obtain personal details from the patient.
2. Explain the importance of giving up smoking.

New words

1. admission / ədˈmɪʃn / *n.* the act of admitting someone to enter 入院
2. next of kin: the person who is your closest relative, especially in official or legal documents 最近的亲人
3. occupation / ɒkjʊˈpeɪʃn / *n.* a job or profession 职业
4. inform / ɪnˈfɔːm / *vt.* to officially tell someone about something or give them information 通知；告知
5. receptionist / rɪˈsepʃənɪst / *n.* someone whose job is to welcome and deal with people arriving in a hotel or office building, visiting a doctor etc. 前台接待
6. consult / kənˈsʌlt / *vt.* to ask for information or advice from someone 咨询；请教
7. pharmacy / ˈfɑːməsi / *n.* the science and technique of preparing and dispensing drugs and medicines 配药学
8. ward / wɔːd / *n.* a suite of rooms shared by patients who need a similar kind of care 病房
9. surgery / ˈsɜːdʒəri / *n.* the branch of medical science that treats disease or injury by operative procedures 外科
10. emergency room: a room in a hospital or clinic staffed and equipped to provide emergency care to persons requiring immediate medical treatment 急诊室
11. kidney / ˈkɪdni / *n.* either of the two bean-shaped excretory organs that filter wastes (especially urea) from the blood and excrete them and water in urine 肾脏
12. diabetes / ˌdaɪəˈbiːtiːz / *n.* any of the several metabolic disorders marked by excessive urination and persistent thirst 糖尿病
13. endocrine / ˈendəʊkrɪn / *adj.* relating to the system in your body that produces hormones 内分泌的
14. pulmonary / ˈpʌlmənəri / *adj.* relating to or affecting the lungs 肺的
15. manual / ˈmænjuəl / *adj.* of or relating to the hands; doing or requiring physical work 手工的；

靠劳力的

16. ruptured / 'rʌptʃə(r)d / *adj.* suddenly and violently broken open especially from internal pressure 破裂的

17. pediatrics / ˌpiːdi'ætrɪks / *n.* the branch of medicine concerned with the treatment of infants and children 儿科

18. maternity / mə'tɜːnəti / *n.* the period from conception to birth when a woman carries a developing fetus in her uterus 孕产期

19. geriatrics / dʒeri'ætrɪks / *n.* the branch of medical science that deals with diseases and problems specific to old people 老年病科

20. radiology / ˌreɪdi'ɒlədʒi / *n.* the branch of medical science dealing with the medical use of X-rays or other penetrating radiation 放射线科

21. midwife / 'mɪdwaɪf / *n.* a woman skilled in aiding the delivery of babies 助产士

22. pajamas / pə'dʒɑːməz / *n.* (usually plural) loose-fitting nightclothes worn for sleeping or lounging 睡衣

23. originally / ə'rɪdʒɪnəli / *adv.* with reference to the origin or beginning 最初地

24. gender / 'dʒendə(r) / *n.* the fact of being male or female 性别

25. marital / 'mærɪtl / *adj.* of or relating to the state of marriage 婚姻的

26. widow / 'wɪdəʊ / *n.* a woman whose husband has died and who has not married again 寡妇；遗孀

27. bracelet / 'breɪslət / *n.* a band of cloth or leather or metal links attached to a wristwatch and wrapped around the wrist 手环

28. allergy / 'ælədʒi / *n.* hypersensitivity reaction to a particular allergen; symptoms can vary greatly in intensity 过敏症

29. blood pressure / blʌd preʃə(r) / *n.* the amount of force with which your blood flows around your body 血压

30. bronchitis / brɒŋ'kaɪtɪs / *n.* an illness like a very bad cough, in which your bronchial tubes become sore and infected 支气管炎

Taking Vital Signs

Intended Learning Objectives

On completion of the unit, students should be able to:

1. describe vital signs;
2. describe readings;
3. take vital signs using appropriate English to communicate with patients;
4. report vital signs to other medical professionals.

Lead-in

Listen and repeat. 🎧

Listen to the following sentences and repeat them. Pay attention to the pronunciation and intonation.

1. I'm just going to do your observations, is that OK?
2. Mr. Blake in bed 301 is now in rapid AF (atrial fibrillation). Can you please put him onto hourly obs. ?
3. Please put this thermometer under your armpit for a short while, and keep your arm firmly up against your chest until I take it out.
4. The normal range for the body temperature is around 36 to 37 ℃.
5. I'm just going to take your pulse. Can I have your wrist, please?
6. Hello Betty, Paul Miller in bed 15 is quite tachycardic. His heart rate is 130 but he is still in a regular sinus rhythm.
7. Before I take your blood pressure, could you please tell me if you have had any previous surgery done on either your chest or arms?
8. When I inflate the blood pressure cuff, it'll be a little tight.
9. His Resps. (respirations) were 18 at 14: 00.
10. Mrs. Chan still remains quite tachypnoeic most of the time, at a rate of 35.

Communication Focus

A patient's consent must be obtained before a nurse performs any healthcare procedures.

In pairs, discuss the following questions.

1. Why do you think obtaining a patient's consent is important?
2. How do you acquire the consent?

Part One   Describing Vital Signs

Task 1 **Work in pairs.**

Match the abbreviations on the chart to the words below. Explain the abbreviations to your partner.

Example: BP stands for; BP means…

Observation Chart

Patient name: Phillip Bracknell

Date/Time	BP	P	RR	T	Wt.	O₂Sat	Signature
15/12/2014 8: 00 a. m.	130/90	78	14	37.5	75kg	95%	R. Perez

1. kilogram _____
3. respiratory rate _____
5. temperature _____
7. blood pressure_____

2. percent _____
4. pulse _____
6. oxygen saturation _____
8. weight _____

Task 2 **Pronounce the words.** 🎧

Write down the words according to the phonetic symbols below. And then listen and check.

1. / hɑːt reɪt / _____
3. / blʌd preʃə(r) / _____
5. / 'temprətʃə(r) / _____
7. / ˌsætʃə'reɪʃn / _____

2. / pʌls / _____
4. / rə'spɪrətri / _____
6. / 'ɒksɪdʒən / _____
8. / ˌɒbzə'veɪʃn / _____

Task 3 **Read aloud and check.** 🎧

Read the following measurements and put a tick (√) in the correct column. And then listen to the audio and check.

		RR	BP	P	T
1	135mmHg				
2	36.7 ℃				
3	75bpm				
4	20bpm				
5	98.6°F				

Part Two   Monitoring Vital Signs

Task 4 **Work in pairs.**

Label the pictures of medical instruments with the words below. And describe what each piece of equipment is used to measure.

Example: A stethoscope is used to monitor/measure...

A watch with second hand is used when...

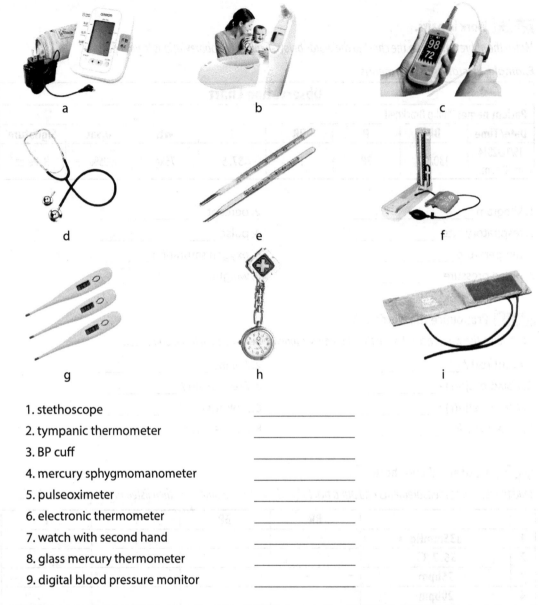

a

b

c

d

e

f

g

h

i

1. stethoscope   _____
2. tympanic thermometer   _____
3. BP cuff   _____
4. mercury sphygmomanometer   _____
5. pulseoximeter   _____
6. electronic thermometer   _____
7. watch with second hand   _____
8. glass mercury thermometer   _____
9. digital blood pressure monitor   _____

Note:

Different ways of taking temperature—by mouth (oral temperature); by armpit (axillary temperature); by rectum (rectal temperature); by ear (tympanic/ear temperature)

Task 5 Work in pairs. 🎧

Put these words in order to make sentences. Discuss which vital sign the nurse is taking in each case. Listen and check your answers.

1. hold, me, arm, you, your, Can, for, straight, out?

2. tongue, this, pop, Just, your, under.

3. ear, into, I'll, this, your, probe, put.

4. have, I, wrist, please, Can, your?

5. roll, your, Can, up, you, sleeve?

6. finger, into, Please, put, probe, your, this.

7. and, out, in, Just, normally, breathe.

8. me, you, hand, Can, right, give, please, your?

Task 6 Role-play. 🎧

Play the role and listen to the sample.

Scenario: in the admitting room

Instruments needed: a thermometer, a sphygmomanometer, a watch with second hand, and an obs. chart

Task: Student A plays as a nurse to take vital signs for student B. And swap the role later.

Useful sentence patterns:

1. Did you drink any hot water in the last half an hour?

2. Have you been smoking, drinking coffee or taking any kind of stimulants today?

3. Do you have any history of high blood pressure?

4. Please give me the thermometer.

5. Lift your arm a little so I can put on the blood pressure cuff.

6. How is my pulse?

7. Do I have a temperature?

8. I'll report all the results to the doctor.

Part Three   Reporting Vital Signs

Task 7 Work in pairs. 🎧

Look at the graphs and try to describe the changes of vital signs. In the graphs, the unit for each vital sign has been deliberately omitted. So the students should first recognize it and decide which sign the graph is about. And then listen to the audio and match each graph to the patient.

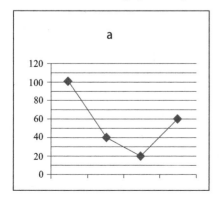

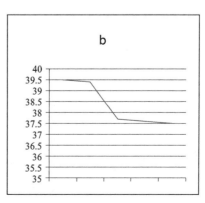

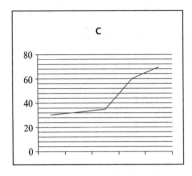

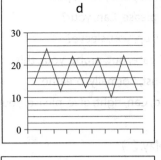

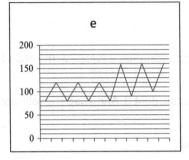

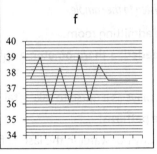

1. Patient 1 _____   2. Patient 2 _____
3. Patient 3 _____   4. Patient 4 _____
5. Patient 5 _____   6. Patient 6 _____

Note:

1. ↗ increase/rise/go up
2. ↘ decrease/fall/go down
3. ⌒ go up and down/vary between … and …
4. — be stable/remain the same/settle
5. ∿ go up and down/vary between … and…

(We usually use simple past tense to report the readings of vital signs.)

Task 8 **Listen and complete.** 🎧

Listen to the audio and complete the chart. And act it out in pairs.

Observation Chart					U / N: 201984 Surname: Carter Given names: Felton DOB: 22 / 9 / 1945 Sex: Male		
Date	**Time**	**T**	**P**	**R**	**BP**	**Comment**	**Signature**
2/3/2017	02：00	1.	2.	18	3.		J. Perez
2/3/2017	06：00	36. 4	4.	16	5.		J. Perez
2/3/2017	10：00	36. 4	6.	7.	8.		J. Perez
2/3/2017	14：00	36. 3	9.	20	10.		J. Perez
2/3/2017	15：00	36. 5	11.	18	12.		J. Perez

Observation Chart						U / N: 201975 Surname: Castle Given names: Rosa DOB: 9 / 2 / 1968 Sex: Female		

Date	Time	T	P	R	BP	Comment	Signature
2/3/2017	06: 00	37. 3	72	13. ___	130/90		J. Perez
2/3/2017	07: 00	37. 5	76	18	105/65		J. Perez
2/3/2017	08: 00					OT	J. Perez
2/3/2017	09: 00					OT	J. Perez
2/3/2017	10: 00					OT	J. Perez
2/3/2017	11: 00					OT	J. Perez
2/3/2017	12: 00					OT	J. Perez
2/3/2017	13: 00					OT	J. Perez
2/3/2017	14: 00	37. 2	78	14. ___	120/75		J. Perez
2/3/2017	15: 00	37. 4	76	15. ___	115/65		J. Perez

Task 9 **Practice.**

Read the following chart and practice handing over the patient Gladys Small.

Observation Chart						U / N: 29034 Surname: Small Given Names: Gladys Bed No. : 32 DOB: 25 / 9 / 1977 Sex: Female	

Date	Time	T	P	R	BP	Comment	Signature
8/11/2017	07: 00	38. 9	100	18	170/110		J. R. Pland(RN)
8/11/2017	12: 35	37. 9	90	18	200/120	IV given as ordered	J. R. Pland(RN)
8/11/2017	15: 00	37. 2	86	18	140/90		J. R. Pland(RN)

More Practice

Role-play.

Read the following case and play the roles of a nurse and a patient based on the case. In the dialogue, you should complete the tasks below the case.

> **Case Study:** Mr. Ford is a 32-year-old man who works as a physical trainer at the local gym. He has been admitted to the A&E unit following a knee injury sustained during a gym session. You are asked to obtain personal details from the patient and to assess and record his vital signs. His temperature and respirations are fine but his pulse is only 48 bpm. He appears to be well, apart from his painful knee.

Tasks:

1. Find out the reasons for the abnormality of the vital signs.
2. Explain the abnormality and comfort the patient.

New words

1. observation / ˌɒbzəˈveɪʃ(ə)n / *n.* something that you notice when watching something or someone 观察结果

2. atrial / ˈeɪtriəl / *adj.* of or relating to a cavity or chamber in the body (especially one of the upper chambers of the heart) 心房的

3. fibrillation / ˌfaɪbrɪˈleɪʃən / *n.* a local and uncontrollable twitching of muscle fibres, esp. of the heart, not affecting the entire muscle 纤维性颤动

4. thermometer / θəˈmɒmɪtə(r) / *n.* a piece of equipment that measures the temperature of the air, of your body etc. 温度计；体温计

5. armpit / ˈɑːmpɪt / *n.* the hollow place under your arm where it joins your body 腋窝

6. Celsius / ˈselsiəs / *n.* a scale of temperature in which water freezes at 0° and boils at 100° 摄氏度

7. wrist / rɪst / *n.* the part of your body where your hand joins your arm 腕（关节）

8. tachycardic / ˌtækɪˈkɑːdɪk / *adj.* of or relating to abnormally rapid beating of the heart, esp. over 100 beats per minute 心动过速的；心搏过速的

9. sinus / ˈsaɪnəs / *n.* the hollow spaces in the bones of the head that are connected to the inside of the nose 窦；窦房结

10. inflate / ɪnˈfleɪt / *v.* to fill something with air or gas so it becomes larger, or to become filled with air or gas（使）充气；（使）膨胀

11. tachypnoeic / ˌtækɪpˈniːik / *adj.* of or relating to abnormally rapid breathing 呼吸过速的

12. respiratory / rəˈspɪrətri / *adj.* relating to breathing 呼吸的

13. saturation / ˌsætʃəˈreɪʃn / *n.* the degree to which something has been mixed into something else 饱和度

14. mercury / ˈmɜːkjəri / *n.* a heavy silver-white poisonous metal that is liquid at ordinary temperatures, and is used in thermometers 水银；汞

15. stethoscope / ˈsteθəskəʊp / *n.* an instrument that a doctor uses to listen to your heart or breathing 听诊器

16. tympanic / tɪmˈpænɪk / *adj.* of or relating to the main cavity of the ear which is between the eardrum and the inner ear 鼓膜的；耳膜的

17. sphygmomanometer / ˌsfɪgməʊməˈnɒmɪtə / *n.* a pressure gauge for measuring blood pressure 血压计

18. pulse oximeter / ˌpʌls ɒkˈsɪmɪtə / *n.* a device attached to a fingertip to monitor the amount of oxygen carried in the body and the heart rate 脉氧仪

19. axillary / ækˈsɪləri / *adj.* of, relating to, or near the armpit 腋窝的；靠近腋窝的

20. rectum / ˈrektəm / *n.* the final straight portion of the large intestine 直肠

21. probe / prəʊb / *n.* a long thin metal instrument that doctors and scientists use to examine parts

of the body 探针

22. stimulant / ˈstɪmjələnt / n. a drug or substance that makes you feel more active and full of energy 兴奋剂；引起兴奋的物质

23. hypertension / haɪpəˈtenʃn / n. a medical condition in which your blood pressure is too high 高血压

24. hypertensive / ˌhaɪpəˈtensɪv / adj. having abnormally high blood pressure 高血压的

25. ECG: electrocardiogram / ɪˌlektrəʊˈkɑːdiəʊgræm / n. the recording of the electrical activity of the heart 心电图

26. GTN: glyceryl trinitrate / ˈɡlɪs(ə)raɪl ˈtraɪˈnaɪtreɪt / n. a medication used for heart failure, high blood pressure, and to treat and prevent chest pain from not enough blood flow to the heart (angina) or due to cocaine 硝酸甘油

27. sublingually / sʌbˈlɪŋɡwəlɪ / adv. by the means of putting beneath the tongue 舌下给药

28. pre-op: preoperative / priˈɒpərətɪv / adj. relating to the time before a medical operation 手术前的

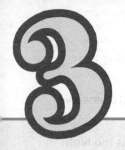

Researching Symptoms

Intended Learning Objectives

On completion of the unit, students should be able to:

1. describe symptoms;
2. ask about symptoms of illnesses and injuries;
3. research symptoms using appropriate English to communicate with patients;
4. report symptoms to other medical professional.

Lead-in

Listen and repeat. 🎧

Listen to the following sentences and repeat them. Pay attention to the pronunciation and intonation.

1. What seems to be the trouble?
2. Please show me where the pain is.
3. Do you feel short of breath and are there any changes in your vision?
4. Does the pain spread anywhere else?
5. Have you had any nausea and vomiting?
6. How about your bowel movement? And have you been passing any wind?
7. Have you noticed any blood in your motions/in your sputum/when you pass water?
8. Do you get a pain in your chest when you cough?
9. Have you noticed any coffee grounds, bile and blood in your vomit?
10. Did you run a fever or have a sore throat?

Communication Focus

There are two major linguistic challenges you will face working as a nurse in a native English-speaking healthcare context: Mastering laypersons' healthcare English; Mastering professional healthcare English (medical terms).

In pairs, discuss how to correct the ineffective communication sentences.

1. RN: We are going to give you thrombolysis for your infarct now.
2. RN: We are going to start you on a heparin infusion now. It's an IV anticoagulant.

Part One Describing Symptoms

Task 1 **Work in pairs.** 🎧

Look at the following pictures and try to describe the symptoms. And then listen to the 10 patients describing their symptoms and match them to the pictures a-j.

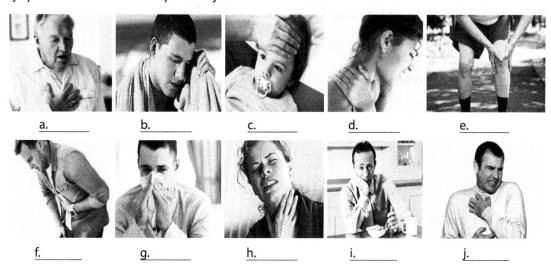

a._____   b._____   c._____   d._____   e._____

f._____   g._____   h._____   i._____   j._____

Work in small groups. Choose five symptoms among those in task 1 that you think they are the main reasons for patients to see a doctor in China. And then give the reasons.

Example: *I think … is among the top five symptoms because…*

Task 2 **Work in pairs.** 🎧

Match 1-5 to a-e to make questions. Then listen and check your answer.

1. How long have   a. moved again?

2. Has it   b. you had the pain in your belly?

3. Does the characteristic   c. of the pain change?

4. Have you had   d. have a fever ?

5. Did you   e. any diarrhea?

Task 3 **Read and complete.**

Read the answers the patient gave to the nurse. Write the nurse's questions.

1. N:_____?

   P: Since last night, it started around the umbilicus, but moved to the right this morning.

2. N:_____?

   P: No. It has been steady for 4 hours.

3. N:_____?

   P: It started as a blunt pain, but changed to a sharp pain, so severe that I can hardly stand it.

4. N:_____?

    P: No. I haven't had any bowel movement for 2 days.

5. N:_____?

    P: Last night I took my temperature. It was 38 degrees Celsius.

Part Two　Inquiring About Symptoms

Task 4 Work in pairs.

Look at the patient in this photo. Work in pairs and discuss the following questions.

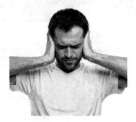

1. What are the patient's symptoms?

2. What's the patient suffering from?

3. What do you think he should do?

Task 5 Listen and complete. 🎧

Listen to the nurse interviewing Mr. Smith and check your answers in Task 4. Listen again and complete the patient record.

Peking University People's Hospital **Patient Record**
Patient: Mr. Smith　　　　**Age:** 40 **DOA:** 20/7/2017
Problems: He has pains in the 1._____ and is suffering from 2._____ . The pain is concentrated on the 3._____ , accompanied by 4._____ in the morning. The patient noticed a blurring of 5._____ and saw 6._____ three times. But there is no trouble with his 7._____ . These days before he has had a fit, he felt 8._____ . His 9._____ is worse than ever. He is also suffering from 10._____ in his limbs.

Task 6 Role-play. 🎧

Play the role and listen to the sample.

Scenario: in the consulting room

Instruments needed: a thermometer, a tongue depressor, a penlight, a blood taking needle and chart

Task: Student A plays as a nurse to ask student B, mother of the patient, about the symptoms of her child. The child is likely to have a scarlet fever. Student C plays as the child. And swap the role later.

Useful sentence patterns:

1. My child has a temperature, a headache, a sore throat and a rash.

2. How long has he been ill?

3. Are there any sick children in the neighborhood or at school?

4. Let me have a look. Open your mouth and show me your tongue. Now take off your clothes.

5. His tonsils are swollen and red. His tongue is as red as a strawberry. There is a rash all over his body.

6. He may need a blood test.

7. Here is the result. Is it normal?

8. His white blood cell count is high. He is probably suffering from scarlet fever.

9. It is a kind of infectious disease. You should keep him away from other children as much as possible.

10. Does he need to take some drugs?

Part Three   Reporting Symptoms

Task 7 Work in pairs.

Read this report about a patient suffering from a car accident and find four mistakes.

Last night Miss Miller had a car accident and bled a lot. She had lost consciousness for a while. Later she was admitted to the hospital and was given an injection of 5ml tetanus toxoid by the nurse. Today she is not feeling any pain. She is supposed to be supported by the cast and body with pillows in good alignment and keep the cast uncovered. Any sign of decreased circulation, coldness, swelling or numbness should be reported.

Task 8 Practice.

Report this patient who has appendicitis to the head nurse using these notes.

Patient name: Mr. Williams

History:

Yesterday—a mild fever, a loss of appetite, suffering from nausea, vomiting with an occasional pain in the center of his stomach

On admission—severe abdominal pain

This morning—swollen abdomen, suffering from a constant sharp pain in his lower right side

Research the symptoms of one of these illnesses and give a short presentation describing them to the class.

AIDS

tuberculosis

leprosy

More Practice

Role-play.

Read the following case and play the roles of a nurse and a patient based on the case. In the dialogue, you should complete the tasks below the case.

Case Study: A victim in a road accident got severely injured on his head and was knocked out for a short while on the scene. He was then sent to the emergency department. You are asked to interview him about how it happened and some other related information.

Tasks:

1. Find out the symptoms of the victim in the accident.

2. Provide the treatments and comfort the patient.

New words

1. nausea / ˈnɔːziə / *n.* disgust so strong that it makes you feel sick 恶心

2. bowel movement / ˈbaʊəl ˈmuːvmənt / *n.* the last stop in the movement of food through your digestive tract. Your stool passes out of your body through the rectum and anus 排便

3. sputum / ˈspjuːtəm / *n.* saliva mixed with discharges from the respiratory passages 痰

4. thrombolysis / θrɒmˈbɒlɪsɪs / *n.* the process of breaking up and dissolving blood clots 血栓溶解

5. infarct / inˈfɑːkt / *n.* localized necrosis resulting from obstruction of the blood supply 梗死

6. bile / baɪl / *n.* a digestive juice secreted by the liver and stored in the gallbladder 胆汁

7. coffee grounds / ˈkɒfɪ graʊndz / *n.* the dregs remaining after brewing coffee 咖啡渣

8. renal / ˈriːnl / *adj.* of or relating to the kidneys 肾脏的

9. dietitian / daɪəˈtɪʃn / *n.* a specialist in the study of nutrition 营养学家

10. supplement / ˈsʌplɪmənt / *n.* a quantity added (e. g. to make up for a deficiency) 补充物

11. NG tube: nasogastric tube / neizəuˈgæstrik tjuːb / *n.* a special tube that carries food and medicine to the stomach through the nose 鼻胃管

12. layperson / ˈleɪpɜːsn / *n.* someone who is not a clergyman or a professional person 外行

13. gland / glænd / *n.* any of the various organs that synthesize substances needed by the body and release it through ducts or directly into the bloodstream 腺体

14. diarrhea / daɪəˈrɪə / *n.* frequent and watery bowel movements; can be a symptom of infection or

food poisoning or colitis or a gastrointestinal tumor 腹泻

15. umbilicus / ʌm'bɪlɪkəs / *n.* the small hollow part or lump in the middle of the stomach where the umbilical card was cut at birth 肚脐

16. limb / lɪm / *n.* one of the jointed appendages of an animal used for locomotion or grasping: arm, leg, wing, flipper 四肢

17. scarlet fever / 'skɑːlət͵'fiːvə(r) / *n.* an acute communicable disease (usually in children) characterized by fever and a red rash 猩红热

18. tonsil / 'tɒnsɪl / *n.* either of the two masses of lymphatic tissue, one on each side of the oral pharynx 扁桃体

19. rash / ræʃ / *n.* any red eruption of the skin 皮疹

20. appendicitis / ə͵pendə'saɪtɪs / *n.* inflammation of the vermiform appendix 阑尾炎

21. malaria / mə'leərɪə / *n.* an infective disease caused by sporozoan parasites that are transmitted through the bite of an infected Anopheles mosquito; marked by paroxysms of chills and fever 疟疾

22. leprosy / 'leprəsi / *n.* chronic granulomatous communicable disease occurring in tropical and subtropical regions; characterized by inflamed nodules beneath the skin and wasting of body parts; caused by the bacillus Mycobacterium leprae 麻风病

23. tuberculosis / tjuː͵bɜːkju'ləʊsɪs / *n.* infection transmitted by inhalation or ingestion of tubercle bacilli and manifested in fever and small lesions (usually in the lungs but in various other parts of the body in acute stages) 肺结核

24. tetanus / 'tetənəs / *n.* an acute and serious infection of the central nervous system caused by bacterial infection of open wounds 破伤风

25. toxoid / 'tɒksɔɪd / *n.* a bacterial toxin that has been weakened until it is no longer toxic but is strong enough to induce the formation of antibodies and immunity to the specific disease caused by the toxin 类毒素

Collecting Samples

Intended Learning Objectives

On completion of the unit, students should be able to:

1. name the common medical specimens;
2. describe the common lab tests;
3. collect samples using appropriate English to communicate with patient;
4. report lab tests to other medical professionals.

Lead-in

Listen and repeat. 🎧

Listen to the following sentences and repeat them. Pay attention to the pronunciation and intonation.

1. I will collect your blood to make sure what caused the fever.
2. Please roll up your sleeve, and lay your arm on the table.
3. I will sterilize your skin and tie the tourniquet around your arm.
4. I need to change the specimen tube. Please clench your fist.
5. I'm going to collect your urine to do a urinalysis.
6. I have brought you a urinal—this bottle. Please pass urine into it.
7. Please get some of your stools with this little spoon and put it back into the tube.
8. Please avoid getting any other things into the tube.
9. Otherwise it might give us a false result.
10. I will send the specimen to the lab./I will do the test in the ward. The specimen won't be sent to the lab.

Communication Focus

Nurses should always give relevant explanations and education prior to providing healthcare and they must check to see that education and explanations provided are understood clearly.

In pairs, discuss the following questions.

1. Why do you think explaining and educating in advance is important?
2. How do you make sure that a patient understand you?

Part One　Describing Common Lab Tests and Medical Specimens

Task 1 **Match pictures.**

Match the pictures to the proper names of the test procedures in collecting samples.

Blood Test	Urine Test	Stool (Feces) Test

1. _____ 2. _____ 3. _____

Task 2 **Work in pairs.** 🎧

Listen and match each sample collected with facts as its targets. Then explain the purposes of collecting each sample to your partner.

Example: *The blood will be collected for blood test to look for any sign of … /make sure whether there is a …*

Urine

Blood

Stool (Feces)

a. a problem in the intestine
b. diabetes
c. liver inflammation/hepatitis
d. infection in the bladder
e. infection in the kidneys

Task 3 **Pronounce the words.** 🎧

Write down the words according to the phonetic symbols below. And listen to check.

1. / ˈjʊərɪn / _____
2. / ˌdaɪəˈbiːtiːz / _____
3. / stuːl / _____
4. / ˈfiːsiːz / _____
5. / ɪnˈtestɪn / _____
6. / ɪnˈfekʃn / _____
7. / ˈblædə(r) / _____
8. / ˈkɪdni / _____

Part Two　Helping Patients Collect Samples

Task 4 **Work in pairs.**

Match 1-4 in the illustrations to words a-d. And then describe what they are used to do.

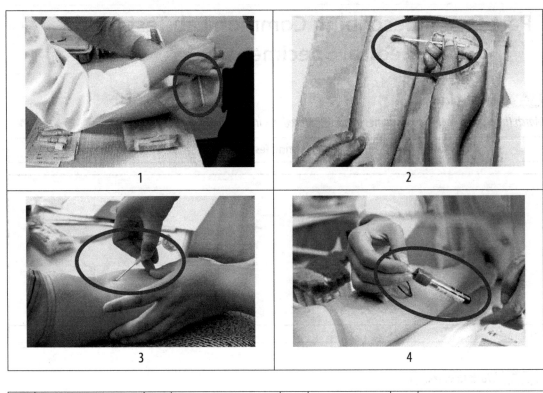

| a. cotton stick | b. tourniquet | c. needle | d. specimen tube |

Task 5 Work in pairs. 🎧

Complete this dialogue about taking a blood sample from a 9 year-old boy with words in Task 4. Then listen and act it out in pairs.

Nurse: Good morning gentlemen. I'm Kelly. I will collect your blood to make sure what caused the fever. You are Calvin Green, right?

Patient: Yes…I don't like blood test! That's painful!

Nurse: If you follow my instructions, I promise, I will do it as gently as I can. Shall we? *(A big smile)*

Patient: …Ok, I will try.

Nurse: Please roll up your sleeve, and lay your arm on the table. I will sterilize your skin. Now I'm going to tie this 1._____ around your arm. Do you feel a small pin prick?

Patient: Yes, it's tight.

Nurse: It won't take long. May I know the name of your school?

(Distracts his attention and inserts the needle.)

Patient: I'm from No. 1 primary school…

Nurse: I see…now I need to change the 2._____. Please clench your fist.

Patient: Oh…I feel dizzy …

Nurse: That will be fine. Be relaxed. Press here with 3._____ for a minute. I will send the specimen to the lab.

Patient: I don't feel well.

Nurse: You may take a rest on the couch. Maybe it will help you.

Patient: Thank you.

Nurse: How do you feel now?

Patient: I feel better. Thank you.

Task 6 Role-play. 🎧

Put these words in 1-16 in the correct order to make sentences and listen to the sentences and check the answer. Then use these sentences to make dialogues about collecting urine or stool and act it out.

Scenario: in the ward

Setting 1: Student A plays as a nurse to collect urine for student B. And swap the role later.

1.	urine/going to/I'm/a/urinalysis/collect/to do/your
2.	in/It can/kidneys/problems/indicate
3.	a urinal/brought you/I have/—this bottle
4.	into/urine/Please/it/pass
5.	dipstick/in the urine specimen/or blood/I will use/sure/a disposable/there is protein/to make
6.	several/It/minutes/only/takes
7.	will/the test/I/ward/do/in/the
8.	sent/The specimen/won't/to the lab/be
9.	ring/ready/it/Please/when/is

Scenario: in the ward

Setting 2: Student A plays as a nurse to collect stool for student B. And swap the role later.

10.	your stool/collect/Next time/we need to/to do a stool test/you open your bowels
11.	It can/in the intestine/indicate/problems
12.	a stool collection tube/Here is/on the lid/with spoon

13.	some of your stools/get/Please/with/into the tube/and put it back/this little spoon
14.	Please avoid/into the tube/getting any other things
15.	a false result/Otherwise/give us/it might
16.	when it is/Please/ring/ready

Part Three   Reporting Lab Tests

Task 7 **Work in pairs.**

Look at the graph and answer the following questions.

<table>
<tr><td colspan="4" align="center">**Complete Blood Count (CBC)**</td></tr>
<tr>
<td colspan="2">**Name:** Eric Naidu
DOB/Sex: 25/3/2000/Male
Ticket No. : 768834021</td>
<td colspan="2">**Date Performed:** 16: 52 7/11/2018
Date Received: 15: 30 7/11/2018
Date Collected: 14: 05 7/11/2018</td>
</tr>
<tr><td align="center">**Test**</td><td align="center">**Result**</td><td align="center">**Unit**</td><td align="center">**Normal Range**</td></tr>
<tr><td>Leukocyte (LEU or WBC = white blood cell)</td><td align="center">13. 40</td><td align="center">$\times 10^9$/L</td><td align="center">4. 0-10. 0</td></tr>
<tr><td align="center">Neutrophil</td><td align="center">9. 40</td><td align="center">$\times 10^9$/L</td><td align="center">2. 0-7. 0</td></tr>
<tr><td>Erythrocyte (ERY or RBC = red blood cell)</td><td align="center">4. 50</td><td align="center">$\times 10^{12}$/L</td><td align="center">3. 5-5. 5</td></tr>
<tr><td align="center">Hemoglobin (Hb or HGB)</td><td align="center">130</td><td align="center">g/L</td><td align="center">110-150 (female)
120-160 (male)</td></tr>
</table>

1. What test was performed?

2. What type of specimen was collected?

3. When was the specimen collected?

4. What time was the specimen analyzed in the lab?

5. How is Eric Naidu's CBC result? Is there anything abnormal?

Task 8 **Listen and complete.** 🎧

Listen to the audio and match the report with the patient.

A. Blood Test			
Test	**Result**	**Unit**	**Normal Range**
Leukocyte	12. 5	$\times 10^9$/L	4. 0-10. 0
Neutrophil	9. 00	$\times 10^9$/L	2. 0-7. 0
Erythrocyte	3. 50	$\times 10^{12}$/L	3. 5-5. 5

Test	Result	Unit	Normal Range
Hemoglobin	130	g/L	110-150 (female) 120-160 (male)

B. Urine Report

Test	Result	Unit	Normal Range
Colour	Light Red	/	/
pH	6. 0	/	4. 5-8. 0
Leukocyte	4+	/	Negative
Protein (PRO)	1+	/	Negative
Occult Blood (OB)	2+	/	Negative

C. Stool (Feces) Report

Physical & Chemical

Stool Colour	Black	Stool Form	Unformed
Test	**Result**	**Unit**	**Normal Range**
Leukocyte	3	HP	0-2
Erythrocyte	3	HP	0-2
Occult Blood	Positive		Negative

Patient 1:		Patient 2:		Patient 3:	

Task 9 Practice in pairs. 🎧

Listen and mark down the professional and laypersons' English for each Chinese term. Then act it out in pairs. Then practice the task below with your partner.

Roles: Student A acts as A nurse

Student B acts as a patient and a doctor

Scenario 1: A nurse gets the *blood report* in task 8 and tries to acquire more symptoms from the patient and then report to the doctor.

Scenario 2: A nurse gets the *urine report* in task 8 and tries to acquire more symptoms from the patient and then report to the doctor.

Scenario 3: A nurse gets the *stool report* in task 8 and tries to acquire more symptoms from the patient and then report to the doctor.

*Please use proper ways (professional or laypersons' terms) to communicate.

Inter-professional English	Laypersons' English	Chinese
		痰
		尿频
		排尿困难
		尿急
		大便未成形

More Practice

Role-play.

Read the following case and play the roles of a nurse and a patient based on the case. In the dialogue, you should complete the tasks below the case.

Case Study: Mrs. Nelson is a 38-year-old woman who has been married for 8 years. She reports suffering from frequent urination, dysuria and urge incontinence. You are asked to help her collect midstream urine following these steps.

1. Wash her hands thoroughly and clean the area around her urethra with disposable wipes.
2. Take the lid off the specimen container. Don't touch the inside of the container.
3. Pass some urine into the toilet and then pass a small amount of urine into the specimen container. That's the middle part of the stream of urine.
4. Tighten the lid and pass it to the nurse.

Tasks:

1. Explain and educate prior to the midstream urine collection.
2. Ensure that education and explanations provided are understood clearly.

New words

1. fever / ˈfiːvə(r) / *n.* a rise in the temperature of the body; frequently a symptom of infection 发烧
2. sleeve / sliːv / *n.* the part of a garment that is attached at the armhole and that provides a cloth covering for the arm 袖子
3. sterilize / ˈsterəlaɪz / *v.* to make something completely clean by killing any bacteria in it 消毒
4. tourniquet / ˈtʊənɪkeɪ / *n.* a band of cloth that is twisted tightly around an injured arm or leg to stop it bleeding 止血带
5. specimen / ˈspesɪmən / *n.* a small amount or piece that is taken from something, so that it can be tested or examined 标本
6. specimen tube / tjuːb / *n.* a glass tube closed at one end 样本试管
7. clench / klentʃ / *v.* to hold your hands, teeth etc. together tightly, usually because you feel angry or determined 握紧
8. urine / ˈjʊərɪn / *n.* the yellow liquid waste that comes out of the body from the bladder 尿液
9. urinalysis / ˌjʊərɪˈnælɪsɪs / *n.* analysis of the urine to test for the presence of disease by the presence of protein, glucose, ketones, cells, etc. 尿液分析
10. urinal / jʊəˈraɪnl / *n.* a type of toilet for men to urinate into 尿壶
11. spoon / spuːn / *n.* an instrument with a handle and a small bowl or cup-shaped extremity 勺子
12. false / fɔːls / *adj.* not in accordance with the fact or reality 错误的
13. in advance: ahead of time; in anticipation 提前
14. stool / stuːl / *n.* a piece of solid waste from your bowels 粪便

15. feces / ˈfiːsiːz / *n.* solid excretory product evacuated from the bowels 粪便

16. infection / ɪnˈfekʃn / *n.* a disease that affects a particular part of your body and is caused by bacteria or a virus 感染

17. bladder / ˈblædə(r) / *n.* the organ in your body that holds urine (= waste liquid) until it is passed out of your body 膀胱

18. sign / saɪn / *n.* an event, fact etc. that shows that something is happening or that something is true or exists 标志

19. liver / ˈlɪvə(r) / *n.* a large organ in your body that produces bile and cleans your blood 肝脏

20. inflammation / ˌɪnfləˈmeɪʃn / *n.* swelling and pain in part of your body, which is often red and feels hot 炎症

21. hepatitis / ˌhepəˈtaɪtɪs / *n.* a disease of the liver that causes fever and makes your skin yellow. There are several types of hepatitis 肝炎

22. suspect / səˈspekt / *v.* to think that something is probably true, especially something bad 怀疑

23. intestine / ɪnˈtestɪn / *n.* the long tube in your body through which food passes after it leaves your stomach 肠

24. cotton stick / ˈkɒtn stɪk / *n.* something consists of a small wad of cotton wrapped around one or both ends of a short rod, usually made of either wood, rolled paper or plastic 棉签

25. needle / ˈniːdl / *n.* a very thin, pointed steel tube at the end of a syringe, which is pushed into your skin to put a drug or medicine into your body or to take out blood 针头

26. instruction / ɪnˈstrʌkʃn / *n.* a statement telling someone what they must do 指令

27. gently / ˈdʒentli / *adv.* in a gentle way 轻轻地

28. prick / prɪk / *n.* a slight pain you get when something sharp goes into your skin 刺痛

29. insert / ɪnˈsɜːt / *v.* to put something inside or into something else 插入

30. primary school: a school for children in the first five or six years of their education 小学

31. dizzy / ˈdɪzi / *adj.* feeling unable to stand steadily, for example because you are looking down from a high place or because you are ill 头晕的

32. indicate / ˈɪndɪkeɪt / *v.* to show that a particular situation exists, or that something is likely to be true 表明

33. disposable / dɪˈspəʊzəbl / *adj.* intended to be used once or for a short time and then thrown away 一次性的

34. dipstick / ˈdɪpstɪk / *n.* a strip of cellulose chemically impregnated to render it sensitive to protein, glucose, or other substances in the urine 试纸

35. protein / ˈprəʊtiːn / *n.* one of several natural substances that exists in food such as meat, eggs, and beans, and which your body needs in order to grow and remains strong and healthy 蛋白质

36. lab / læb / *n.* a workplace for the conduct of scientific research 实验室

37. bowel / ˈbaʊəl / *n.* the system of tubes inside your body where food is made into solid waste material and through which it passes out of your body 大肠

38. lid / lɪd / *n.* a cover for the open part of a pot, box, or other containers 盖子

39. occult blood: the blood that is not obvious on examination and is from a nonspecific source, with

obscure signs and symptoms 隐血；潜血

40. watery / ˈwɔːtəri / *adj.* full of water or relating to water 水的；水样的

41. phlegm / flem / *n.* the thick yellowish substance produced in your nose and throat 痰；黏液

42. tenacious / təˈneɪʃəs / *adj.* sticking together 黏着力强的

43. purulent / ˈpjʊərələnt / *adj.* containing or producing pus 脓性的

44. leukocyte / ˈluːkəsaɪt / *n.* blood cells that engulf and digest bacteria and fungi; an important part of the body's defense system (also called white blood cell) 白细胞

45. neutrophil / ˈnjuːtrəʊfɪl / *n.* the chief phagocytic leukocyte; stains with either basic or acid dyes 嗜中性粒细胞

46. erythrocyte / ɪˈrɪθrəsaɪt / *n.* a mature blood cell that contains hemoglobin to carry oxygen to the bodily tissues; a biconcave disc that has no nucleus 红细胞

47. hemoglobin / ˌhiːməˈgləʊbɪn / *n.* a hemoprotein composed of globin and heme that gives red blood cells their characteristic colour; function primarily to transport oxygen from the lungs to the body tissues 血红蛋白

48. liter / ˈliːtə(r) / *n.* a metric unit of capacity equal to the volume of 1 kilogram of pure water at 4 degrees centigrade and 760 mm of mercury (or approximately 1.76 pints) 升

49. gram / græm / *n.* the basic unit for measuring weight in the metric system 克

50. RTI: reproductive tract infection / ˌriːprəˈdʌktɪv ˈtrækt ɪnˈfekʃn / *n.* infections that affect the reproductive tract, which is part of the Reproductive System 生殖道感染

51. pee / piː / *vi.* to pass liquid waste from your body 排尿

52. dysuria / dɪsˈjʊəriə / *n.* difficult or painful urination 排尿困难

53. incontinence / inˈkɒntɪnəns / *n.* involuntary urination or defecation 大小便失禁

54. UTI: urinary tract infection / ˈjʊərɪnəri ˈtrækt ɪnˈfekʃn / *n.* an infection that affects part of the urinary tract 泌尿道感染；尿路感染

55. MSU: midstream urine / ˌmɪdˈstriːm ˈjʊərɪn / MSU is tested to confirm the diagnosis of a urine infection 中段尿

56. poop / puːp / *n.* solid waste from the bowels 粪便

Talking About Pain

Intended Learning Objectives

On completion of the unit, students should be able to:

1. describe pain;
2. assess the pain accurately by using pain assessment scale;
3. discuss pain relief using appropriate English to communicate with patients.

Lead-in

Listen and repeat. 🎧

Listen to the following sentences and repeat them. Pay attention to the pronunciation and intonation.

1. How strong is the pain?
2. What's the pain in your shoulder like?
3. When does the pain start/stop?
4. I've brought a pain chart so you can explain your pain a bit better.
5. Does anything make them worse?
6. What makes the pain better?
7. Do you feel anything else wrong when it's there?
8. What does the pain feel like?
9. How often do you get the pain?
10. Can you tell me on a scale of zero to ten what is the worst pain you've had in the last twenty-four hours in each area?

Communication Focus

A patient's physical pain needs to be acknowledged and taken seriously.

In pairs, discuss the following questions.

1. Why do you think using objective and non-judgmental language to assess patient's pain is important?
2. Which one is effective communication when the nurse responds to the patient's complaint?

Scenario A:

Patient: The pain is just so bad, I can't bear it!

Nurse: Yes, John. It sounds really terrible. I'll get some painkillers for you straight away.

Scenario B:

Patient: The pain is just so bad, I can't bear it!

Nurse: You don't look like you are in pain, you'll be all right, be strong.

Part One   Describing Pain

Task 1 Pronounce the words. 🎧

Write down the words according to the phonetic symbols below. And then listen and check.

1. / ˈeɪkɪŋ / _____
2. / ˈstæbɪŋ / _____
3. / ʃɑːp / _____
4. / ˈtɪŋglɪŋ / _____
5. / ˈbɜːnɪŋ / _____
6. / ˈθrɒbɪŋ / _____
7. / ˈtendə(r) / _____
8. / ˈʃuːtɪŋ / _____
9. / dʌl / _____
10. / ˈkɒlɪki / _____

Task 2 Listen and practice. 🎧

Look at the pictures of people in pain. Listen to six short conversations (1-6) and match the pictures(a-f) to the conversations.

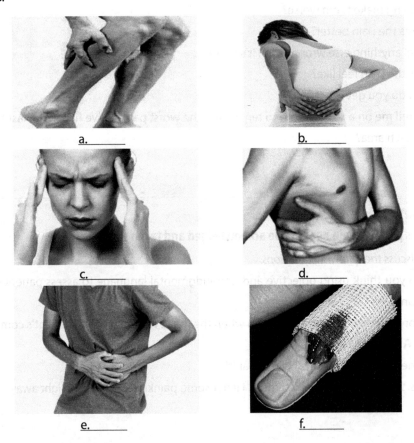

a. _____

b. _____

c. _____

d. _____

e. _____

f. _____

Task 3 Work in pairs. 🎧

Listen to ten patients describing their pain, find out what kind of pain and where the pain is and fill in the table below. Practice describing pain to the medical staff according to the examples as below.

Patient	Type of Pain	Body Part Involved
1		
2		
3		
4		
5		
6		
7		
8		
9		
10		

Practice describing pain to the medical staff according to the examples as below. Use the information in the table above.

Here are some examples of how to describe pain:

Frequency	Impact	Symptom	Body Part
Sometimes	I have trouble walking	from the swelling	in my feet
Every night	I have trouble sleeping	due to the burning pain	in my stomach
Each time	I try to open a bottle, I have trouble twisting the cap	because of stinging pain	in my hands

Part Two   Assessing Pain

Task 4 Recognize pain scales.

A. Match the expressions in the box with the faces and the numbers on the chart.

mild pain; moderate pain; no pain; severe pain; unbearable pain; very severe pain

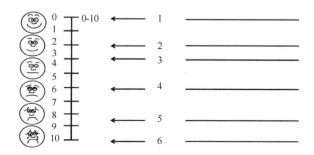

B. Match the words(1-12) and phrases to a question(a-l).

1. Location of the pain	a. How strong is the pain?
2. Pain level	b. When does the pain start?
3. Description of pain (√)	c. When does the pain stop?
4. Trigger	d. Where is the pain?/Where does it hurt?
5. Relivef measure	e. Does anything make them worse?
6. Radiation	f. What makes the pain better? (√)
7. Time of onset	g. Do you feel anything else wrong when it's there?
8. Time of resolution	h. What does the pain feel like?
9. Frequency	i. How often do you get the pain?
10. Aggravation factors	j. How long does the pain last?
11. Associated factors	k. What sets the pain off?
12. Duration	l. Does it go anywhere else?

Task 5 **Listen and practice.** 🎧

Listen to the conversation and fill in the blanks on the Pain Assessment Chart.

Pain Assessment Chart

Patient Name: John
Hospital No. : 3492820

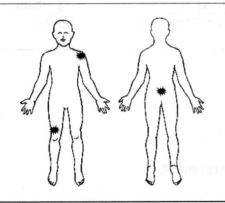

Pain Score
0 1 2 3 4 5 6 7 8 9 10
On a scale of 0-10, what is the worst pain you have had in the last 24 hours?
0 is no pain
1-3 is mild pain
4-6 is moderate pain
7-9 is severe pain
10 is the worst pain imaginable
Record a pain score 0-10 for each site or as mild/moderate/severe if the patient cannot give a number.

Date: 28/2/2018	Pain A	Pain B	Pain C
Location of pain	1.	1.	1.
Pain level	2.	2.	2.
Character	3.	3.	3.
What triggers (starts) the pain?	4.	4.	4.
What relieves the pain (makes the pain better)?	5.	5.	5.

Task 6 Role-play.

In pairs, practice using a Palliative Care Pain Assessment to record a patient's pain. Student A plays as a nurse to assess pain for Student B. Then swap roles and practice again using the Pain Assessment Chart and the patient information below.

Patient Information

The patient's name is Mr. Anthony McGarr. He has advanced cancer of the liver. The pain around his liver is an aching pain, around 5, and is worse when he gets out of bed to walk around. He will feel better when the nurse administers morphine by syringe driver. He also had an infected wound in his right leg. And the pain in the leg is sharp pain. It is 8 and is worse when the dressing is changed. Painkillers before the dressing change and a non-stick dressing make the pain better.

Part Three   Pain Relief

Task 7 Pronounce the words. 🎧

Write down the words according to the phonetic symbols below. And then listen and check.

1. / ˈækjupʌŋktʃə(r) / _____

2. / ˌhɪpnəʊˈθerəpi / _____

3. / ˈmæsɑːʒ / _____

4. / əˌrəʊməˈθerəpi / _____

5. / ˌænəlˈdʒiːziə / _____

6. / ˌhaɪdrəʊˈθerəpi / _____

7. / hiːt pæk / _____

8. / ˈmjuːzɪk ˈθerəpi / _____

9. / ˌkaɪərəʊˈpræktɪk ˈθerəpi / _____

10. / ˈhɜːbl ˈθerəpi / _____

Task 8 Listen and match. 🎧

Some patients choose to use complementary and alternative medicine (CAM) to treat their pain. Look at pictures below. Then listen to the audio about different examples of CAM (1-6) and match the pictures to the types of pain relief (a-f).

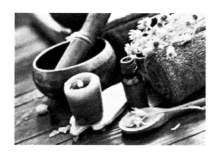

a._____

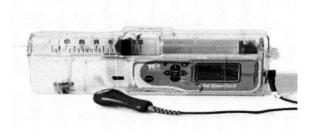

b._____

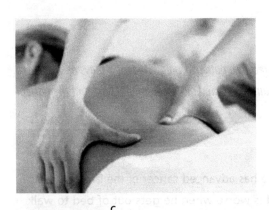

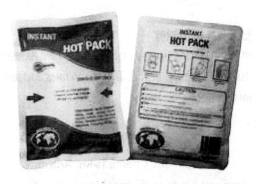

c. _____

d. _____

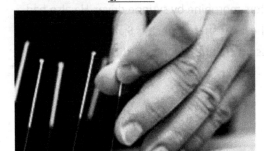

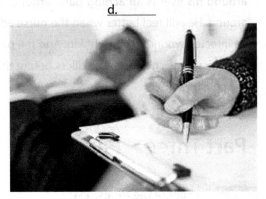

e. _____

f. _____

Task 9 Practice.

In pairs, practice handing over the patient to the next shift. Student A is handing over a patient. Use the information in the box. Student B listens to the handover and makes notes. Swap roles and practice again.

Patient Information

Patient: Jim Sullivan

Bed: 3

Diagnosis: cancer of the liver

Admitted for: palliative care and pain control

Pain: liver pain; an aching pain

Pain Scale: 9 out of 10

Pain relief: a syringe driver will give him a small amount of painkiller medication continuously; heat pack

Review: Doctor Donnely saw him this morning

More Practice

Role-play.

Read the following case and play the roles of a nurse and a patient based on the case. In the dialogue, you should complete the tasks below the case.

Case Study: Charles is a 32-year-old man who has been admitted to orthopedics department for pain control. He was in quite a lot of pain in his knees which lasted for about three to four months. He said the pain would get worse when he stood up. Doctor saw him and ordered a syringe driver. You are asked to assess the pain and explain the reason for pain to the patient.

Tasks:

1. Find out all the information the nurse needs to collect when you assess the pain of the patient.
2. Give some suggestions to the patient to relieve his pain.

New words

1. pain / peɪn / *n.* a symptom of some physical hurt or disorder 疼痛
2. shoulder / ˈʃəʊldə(r) / *n.* the part of the body between the neck and the upper arm 肩膀
3. aching / ˈeɪkɪŋ / *n.* a dull persistent (usually moderately intense) pain 隐隐作痛
4. stabbing / ˈstæbɪŋ / *adj.* as physically painful as if caused by a sharp instrument 刺痛的
5. sharp / ʃɑːp / *adj.* keenly and painfully felt; as if caused by a sharp edge or point 锐痛的
6. tingling / ˈtɪŋglɪŋ / *adj.* causing or experiencing a painful shivering feeling as if from many tiny pricks 有麻刺感的
7. burning / ˈbɜːnɪŋ / *adj.* pain that feels hot as if it were on fire 烧灼痛的
8. throbbing / ˈθrɒbɪŋ / *adj.* pounding or beating strongly or violently （有规律地）抽动的，抽痛的
9. tender / ˈtendə(r) / *adj.* sensitive to touch or palpation 触痛的
10. shooting / ˈʃuːtɪŋ / *n.* (of a pain) that seems to travel like lightning from one place to another 剧痛跳窜；放射性（疼痛）的
11. dull / dʌl / *adj.* a pain that is not severe but does not stop 钝痛的
12. colicky / ˈkɒlɪki / *adj.* suffering from excessive gas in the alimentary canal 绞痛的
13. painkiller / ˈpeɪnkɪlə(r) / *n.* a medicine used to relieve pain 止痛药
14. tablet / ˈtæblət / *n.* a dose of medicine in the form of a small pellet 药片
15. acupuncture / ˈækjupʌŋktʃə(r) / *n.* a chinese treatment of pain or disease by inserting the tips of needles at specific points on the skin 针灸
16. analgesia / ˌænəlˈdʒiːziə / *n.* inability to feel pain 无痛
17. massage / ˈmæsɑːʒ / *n.* the action of squeezing and rubbing someone's body, as a way of making them relax or reducing their pain 按摩

18. aromatherapy / ə,rəʊmə'θerəpi / n. a type of treatment which involves massaging the body with special fragrant oil 芳香疗法

19. hypnotherapy / ,hɪpnəʊ'θerəpi / n. the practice of hypnotizing people in order to help them with a mental or physical problem, for example to help them give up smoking 催眠疗法

20. hydrotherapy / haɪdrəʊ'θerəpi / n. a method of treating people with some diseases or injuries by making them swim or do exercises in water 水疗法

21. herbal / 'hɜ:bl / adj. made from or using herbs 草药的

22. music therapy / 'mju:zɪk 'θerəpi / n. a method of using music to improve health or functional outcomes 音乐疗法

23. chiropractic / ,kaɪrəʊ'præktɪk / n. the treatment of injuries by pressing and moving people's joints, especially the spine 脊柱推拿疗法

24. orthopedics / ,ɔ:θə'pi:dɪks / n. the branch of surgery concerned with disorders of the spine and joints and the repair of deformities of these parts 矫形外科术

25. syringe driver / sɪ'rɪndʒ 'draɪvə(r) / n. a small infusion pump used to gradually administer small amount of fluid to a patient 注射泵

26. trigger / 'trɪgə(r) / n. an act that sets in motion some course of events 诱发因素

Administering Medicine

Intended Learning Objectives

On completion of the unit, students should be able to:

1. explain how to take medication;
2. assist patients with medication according to medication labels;
3. do a medication check and check medication orders for accuracy.

Lead-in

Listen and repeat. 🎧

Listen to the following sentences and repeat them. Pay attention to the pronunciation and intonation.

1. Sally Taylor needs to take 10 milligrams of Zocor once a day by mouth, at bedtime for 90 days.
2. I've got your discharge medication here, Derrick. I just need to explain a few things to you.
3. This one is your antibiotic. Make sure you take it on an empty stomach.
4. The last one is the lotion for your rash. It's important that you shake the bottle so you mix the contents well.
5. Here are the eye drops. They only last a month so remember to discard the contents after this date.
6. Crosscheck the name of the medication on the Prescription Chart and the medication label.
7. I'm going to follow the "five rights" of the medication administration for patient safety.
8. Yes, that's the correct drug, but it should have been ordered by its generic name, furosemide, not its brand name, Lasix.
9. I don't have the right to administer medication without a clear order.
10. Can you see the label to check the dose?

Communication Focus

Healthcare communication should be personalized.

In pairs, discuss the following questions.

1. How do you address a patient to make him/her feel respected as the unique individual?
2. What topics should you choose when you are chatting with patients to add a "personal touch" to your communication?

Part One   Describing Medicine and Medication Route

Task 1 Pronounce the words. 🎧

Work in pairs, match words in the box to pictures a-k. And read after the audio.

inhaler	capsule	suppository	syrup	ointment	injection
tablet	powder	solution	drop	spray	

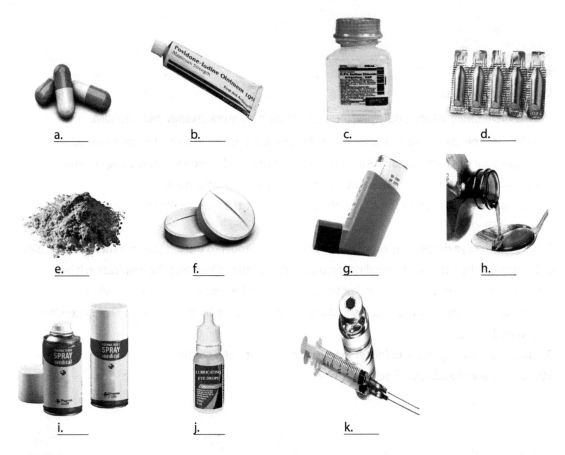

a.＿＿＿　　b.＿＿＿　　c.＿＿＿　　d.＿＿＿

e.＿＿＿　　f.＿＿＿　　g.＿＿＿　　h.＿＿＿

i.＿＿＿　　j.＿＿＿　　k.＿＿＿

Task 2 Work in pairs.

Match the terms and abbreviations (1-14) to the expressions (a-n).

1. qd	a. milligram—unit of mass which is 1/1000 of a gram
2. bid	b. milliliter—unit of volume which is 1/1000 of a litre
3. tid	c. microgram—unit of mass which is 1/1000 of a milligram
4. qid	d. once a day
5. mg	e. three times a day
6. mcg	f. four times a day
7. ml	g. twice a day
8. qod	h. every other day

9. 6/24	i. every six hours
10. IM	j. intravenous injection
11. IV	k. subcutaneous injection
12. SC	l. intradermal injection
13. ID	m. by mouth
14. PO	n. intramuscular injection

Task 3 Listen and complete. 🎧

In pairs, read the prescription and write them out in words. Then listen and check your answer. Practice explaining orders in turns.

Example of prescription:

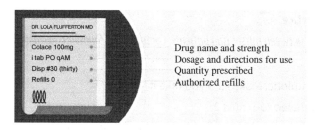

1. Pt: Sally Taylor	2. Pt: Edna Cuthbert	3. Pt: Masoud Khan
Zocor 10mg one	Diovan 40mg (tabs)	Fluvastatin 20mg (caps)
po daily hs	one po tds (pc/ac)	1bd × 7days
Dispense #90	Dispense #30	Dispense #14

1. Sally Taylor needs to take _____ of Zocor once a day _____, at bedtime for _____.

2. Diovan is for your blood pressure. Edna Cuthbert needs to take _____ of Diovan _____ by mouth, _____ for 30 days.

3. Masoud Khan needs to take _____ of Fluvastatin _____ by mouth for 7 days.

Part Two   Instructing Patient to Take Medication Correctly

Task 4 Work in pairs.

Look at the medication labels (1-10) and find a phrase (a-j) with the following meanings.

Medication label	Explanation
1. Shake well before using.	a. Use the medicine only on your skin.
2. For external use only.	b. Do not take it with alcohol.
3. Take with food or milk.	c. Keep it in the fridge between 2−8℃.
4. Contraindications: pregnancy and lactation.	d. Clean the mouth with a mouthful of water.

Medication label	Explanation
5. Do not drink alcoholic beverage.	e. Take all of the medicines for the full length as prescribed by the doctor.
6. Avoid sun exposure.	f. Do not place it directly in the sun.
7. Refrigerate, do not freeze.	g. Shake the bottle thoroughly before you use it.
8. Take on an empty stomach.	h. Do not use it if you are pregnant, or you are likely to be pregnant, or you are breast-feeding your baby.
9. Rinse mouth with water.	i. Take it before eating or drinking.
10. Complete the course of medication.	j. Take the medicine when you are eating or drinking milk.

Task 5 Listen and practice. 🎧

Listen to two conversations between nurses and patients. Complete the following extracts from the conversations.

Conversation 1

This one is your antibiotic. Make sure you take it 1._____.

Now, this is your inhaler. You must 2._____ after you use it.

The last one is the lotion for your rash. It's important that you 3._____ so you mix the contents well.

Conversation 2

Here are the eye drops. They only last a month so remember to 4._____

Don't forget to keep the eye drops 5._____.

You must 6._____ with these tablets. They could burn easily.

Task 6 Work in pairs. 🎧

Practice giving precautions about medications according to your professional knowledge. Use the medication labels in task 4 and the phrases in the box below. And then listen to the audio and repeat.

Don't forget	It's important that	Make sure
Remember to	You must	

Part Three   Administering Medication Correctly

Task 7 Work in pairs.

Look at the "five rights" and discuss their meanings.

> *The Five Rights of Medication Administration*
>
> - Right patient
> - Right medication
> - Right dose
> - Right route
> - Right time

Task 8 **Listen and practice.** 🎧

Jenny, a Student Nurse, is doing a medication check with Joan, a Registered Nurse. Listen to the conversation and mark the order in which Jenny checks the five rights.

Task 9 **Work in pairs.**

Practice checking the medication chart with another nurse. Remember to crosscheck all of the information. Swap roles and practice again.

Patient's name: Mr. Zelnic   U/N: 133579   Bed No. : 1

Name of medication	Route of medication	Dose of medication	Time to be given
warfarin	PO	5mg (one tablet)	16: 00

Useful sentence patterns:

1. Would you mind checking the medication for my patient with me now?

2. What's the medication you need to check?

3. That's what's written here.

4. What time is it due?

5. I'll sign the medication chart first.

6. Let me counter sign for you.

More Practice

Role-play.

Read the following case and play the roles of a nurse and a patient based on the case. In the dialogue, you should complete the tasks below the case.

Case Study: Joan is a 55-year-old female who was transported to the ward after recovering from a surgical procedure. An epidural catheter with morphine was placed for post-operative pain control. Upon arrival, the patient complained of nausea and a headache prompting the on-call physician to prescribe "Demerol 75mg po every three hours for pain". You are asked to administer medication to Joan.

Tasks:

1. Do a medication check before administering.

2. Explain the details of medication to the patient for safety.

New words

1. capsule / ˈkæpsjuːl / *n.* a pill in the form of a small rounded gelatinous container with medicine inside 胶囊

2. inhaler / ɪnˈheɪlə(r) / *n.* a dispenser that produces a chemical vapor to be inhaled in order to relieve nasal congestion 吸入器

3. ointment / ˈɔɪntmənt / *n.* semisolid preparation (usually containing a medicine) applied externally as a remedy or for soothing an irritation 药膏

4. suppository / səˈpɒzətri / *n.* a small plug of medication designed for insertion into the rectum or vagina where it melts 栓剂

5. syrup / ˈsɪrəp / *n.* a thick sweet sticky liquid 糖浆

6. powder / ˈpaʊdə(r) / *n.* any of various cosmetic or medical preparations dispensed in the form of tiny loose particles 药粉

7. solution / səˈluːʃn / *n.* a homogeneous mixture of two or more substances; frequently (but not necessarily) a liquid solution 溶液

8. drop / drɒp / *n.* a small indefinite quantity (especially of a liquid) 液滴

9. injection / ɪnˈdʒekʃn / *n.* the act of putting a liquid into the body by means of a syringe 注射

10. spray / spreɪ / *n.* a dispenser that turns a liquid (such as perfume) into a fine mist 喷雾器

11. milligram / ˈmɪligræm / *n.* one thousandth (1/1, 000) gram 毫克

12. milliliter / ˈmɪliliːtə(r) / *n.* a metric unit of volume equal to one thousandth of a liter 毫升

13. microgram / ˈmaɪkrəʊgræm / *n.* one millionth (1/1, 000, 000) gram 微克

14. intravenous / ˌɪntrəˈviːnəs / *adj.* within or by means of a vein 静脉内的

15. subcutaneous / ˌsʌbkjuˈteɪniəs / *adj.* relating to or located below the epidermis 皮下的

16. intradermal / ˌɪntrəˈdɜːməl / *adj.* relating to areas between the layers of the skin 皮内的

17. intramuscular / ˌɪntrəˈmʌskjələ(r) / *adj.* within a muscle 肌肉内的

18. warfarin / ˈwɔːfərɪn / *adj.* an anticoagulant (trade name Coumadin) used to prevent and treat a thrombus or embolus 华法林

19. dispense / dɪˈspens / *vt.* administer or bestow, as in small portions 分发；发药

20. dose / dəʊs / *n.* a measured portion of medicine taken at any one time 一剂；一服

21. antibiotic / ˌæntibaɪˈɒtɪk / *n.* a chemical substance derivable from a mold or bacterium that kills microorganisms and cures infections 抗生素

22. rinse / rɪns / *vt.* to wash one's mouth and throat with mouthwash 漱口

23. prescription / prɪˈskrɪpʃn / *n.* a piece of paper on which a doctor writes what medicine a sick person should have, so that they can get it from a pharmacist 处方

24. generic / dʒəˈnerɪk / name *adj.* relating to or common to or descriptive of all members of a genus 一般的；通用的

25. furosemide / fjʊəˈrəʊsəmaɪd / *n.* commonly used as diuretic (trade name Lasix) to treat hypertension and edema 利尿剂

Giving IV

Intended Learning Objectives

On completion of the unit, students should be able to:

1. master some abbreviations and terms related to IV administration;
2. describe the administration of IV solution simply;
3. use appropriate English to communicate with patient when giving IV;
4. read and report the charts and documents about IV accurately;
5. master the skills of taking telephone messages accurately and clearly.

Lead-in

Listen and repeat. 🎧

Listen to the following sentences and repeat them. Pay attention to the pronunciation and intonation.

1. The cannula hurts a lot and the IV's not dripping any more.
2. You've still got six doses of IV antibiotics so we need to put a new line.
3. Every time you lifted your arm the infusion stopped.
4. It means inflammation of the vein. More often than not it's caused by a nosocomial infection of staph, originating in hospital.
5. That's why we check the cannula site and take the cannula out at the first sign of infection.
6. She's got an eight hourly litre of normal saline up.
7. Here is her hospital label... Mabyn Hadfield... unit number 62388... date of birth 12th January, 1920.
8. One litre of normal saline over eight hours.
9. The date is 30th of May, the route is IV and the fluid is five percent Dextrose.
10. The rate is one litre over ten hours. That's easy to work out. One litre—a thousand mls—divided by ten hours.

Communication Focus

Non-verbal communication is often more important than verbal communication.

In pairs, discuss the following questions.

1. Why is non-verbal communication often more important than verbal communication?
2. What are the common non-verbal communication modes?

Part One   Preparing for IV

Task 1 **Work in pairs.**

Match Column A with Column B. Explain the abbreviations to your partner.

Example: IV stands for...; IV means...

Column A	Column B
1. IV	a. hours
2. N/S	b. unit number
3. ABs	c. 1 litre
4. 1L	d. intravenous infusion
5. DPM	e. antibiotics
6. Hrs	f. date of birth
7. IVC	g. normal saline
8. ml	h. drops per minute
9. U/N	i. millilitre
10. DOB	j. intravenous cannula

Task 2 **Recognize and read.**

Label the IV equipment (1-6) below using the words in the box. Then read the terms correctly with the audio.

fluid balance chart	IV cannula	IV infusion pump
IV line	IV pole	IV solution

1. _____   2. _____   3. _____

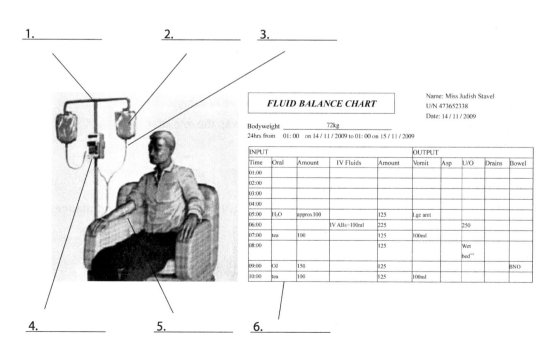

FLUID BALANCE CHART

Name: Miss Judish Stavel
U/N 473652338
Date: 14 / 11 / 2009

Bodyweight _____ 72kg

24hrs from   01: 00   on 14 / 11 / 2009 to 01: 00 on 15 / 11 / 2009

INPUT					OUTPUT				
Time	Oral	Amount	IV Fluids	Amount	Vomit	Asp	U/O	Drains	Bowel
01:00									
02:00									
03:00									
04:00									
05:00	H₂O	approx100		125	Lge amt				
06:00			IV ABs~100ml	225			250		
07:00	tea	100		125	100ml				
08:00				125			Wet bed⁺⁺		
09:00	OJ	150		125					BNO
10:00	tea	100		125	100ml				

4. _____   5. _____   6. _____

Task 3 Read aloud and check. 🎧

Read the following notes and put a tick (√) in the correct column. And then listen to the audio and check.

		Fluid Type	Volume Infused	Drip Rate Calculator	Date/Time	Concentration Percentage
1	1000 ml					
2	30/5 11:00					
3	500ml/hr					
4	167 DPM					
5	5%					
6	normal saline					

Part Two   Administering IV

Task 4 Work in pairs. 🎧

Put these words in order to make sentences. Listen and check your answers.

1. against, IV, Check, physician's, the, solution, orders, the.

2. hands, before, thoroughly, Wash, IV, an, inserting.

3. line, Use, when, sterile, IV, technique, an, inserting.

4. tubing, the, Prime, IV, the, to, system, remove, from, air.

5. being, Label, the, tubing, bags, clearly, and, solution, changed, indicating, when, the, time, date, and.

Task 5 Role-play. 🎧

Listen to the conversation between the nurse and the patient and then play the roles.

Scenario: In the IV Infusion Room.

Instruments needed: an IV pole, IV solution, an IV line, and an IV cannula

Task: Student A plays a nurse to give IV to Student B. And swap the role later.

Useful sentence patterns:

1. It's time to give you intravenous infusion.

2. Could you tell me about the use of the intravenous fluid?

3. The fluid can provide energy for you and prevent you from electrolytic imbalances after operation.

4. Would you please let the fluid drop more quickly?

5. Your intravenous fluid must be given slowly so as not to overload you.

6. Could you help me adjust the air conditioner?

7. Just press the button if you need any help.

8. Sorry to bother you.

Task 6 Listen and match. 🎧

Listen to the audio and match the medical terms (1-9), and then act out the dialogue.

1. nosocomial	a. of the state when an IV line stops running because the line becomes blocked off due to patient's movement
2. phlebitis	b. redness of the skin which can indicate infection
3. infiltration	c. contracted in hospital; from the Greek *noso-*, meaning *disease*
4. staph	d. replace the IV cannula in a different vein
5. IV giving set	e. staphylococci bacteria—types of microbes which are usually found on the skin
6. erythema	f. inflammation of the vein; from the Greek *phleb-*, meaning vein
7. aseptic technique	g. tubing which is spiked into the infusion bag and connected to the IV cannula; also called an IV administration set
8. resite an IV cannula	h. no touch method used to avoid contamination
9. positional	i. condition when fluid leaks into surrounding tissues; in nursing jargon: *tissued*

Part Three   Charting and Documenting About IV

Task 7 Listen and complete. 🎧

Listen to the audio and complete the chart.

IV Prescription Chart	Name of patient: Mabyn Clarke U / N: 62388 DOB: 21 / 1 / 1980 Sex: Female

Fluids must be prescribed daily—only one bag will be administrated against each other

Year: 2019			Medical Officer Prescription			Nursing Administration Record				
Date/ Time	**Line Route**	**Volume**	**Fluid Type and Additive**	**Time to be infused**	**Dr Signature**	**Date Time Start**	**Rate ml/hr**	**Nr1 Nr2**	**Time Stop**	**Volume Infused**
30/5 01: 00	IV	1000ml	Normal Saline	8 hours	H. Khan	30/5 1.____	125ml	G. L V. A	2.____	3.____
30/5 08: 00	5.____	1000ml	6.____ Dextrose	10 hours	H. Khan	4.____ 11: 00	7.____	A. C 8.____		

Task 8 Listen and complete. 🎧

Listen to the audio and circle the details you hear in the chart. And try to practice passing on the message to Michael when he is back.

Date of message	17/9/2018
Time of message	11. 00hrs
Name of caller	Dr. Harris
Nature of call	Resite cannula, Mrs. Blake
Instruction	1. Michael to call Dr. Harris regarding when cannula needs resite 2. Due time next IV ABs 3. Put up another line 4. Bleep Dr. Harris 467
Message documented in Patient Record	Yes/Not necessary
Signature of call recipient	K. Terence (RN)

Note: In order to save time and get all information written down in very short time, in this kind of form, we may use the expressions that maynot be grammatically correct.

Task 9 Role-play.

In pairs, practice giving and taking a telephone message. Student A is a nurse, Rose Williams, from the IV Infusion Room who passes on the messages according to the information in the box; Student B is Jane Smith, a ward nurse who is responsible for taking telephone messages in the chart. Swap roles and practice again.

> Telephone Ward 16C – Mr Henry is booked to have a PICC line inserted tomorrow 10:30 am. He needs a porter to bring him to the IV Infusion Room. Don't forget to bring IV Prescription Chart with him.

Date of message	18/10/2018
Time of message	10.00 hrs
Name of caller	
Nature of call	
Instruction	
Message documented in Patient Record	Yes/Not necessary
Signature of call recipient	

More Practice

Role-play.

Read the following case and play the roles of a nurse and a patient based on the case. In the dialogue, you should complete the tasks below the case.

Case Study: A nurse is preparing to give the medication via IV to Ms. Sara Young, who has been receiving the drug via IV over a number of weeks. And the patient rejects it and says that the physician has agreed to change the mode of administration from IV to oral.

Tasks:

1. Respond to the patient in a positive and friendly way.

2. Use appropriate verbal and non-verbal communication to explain and comfort the patient.

3. Find out whether or not what the patient has said is true.

New words

1. infusion / ɪnˈfjuːʒn / *n.* the act of putting medicine slowly into someone's body, or the medicine itself 注射；注射用药物

2. normal saline: physiological saline, a solution of 0.90% of NaCl, usually used frequently in intravenous drips for patients who cannot take fluids orally and have developed or are in danger of developing dehydration or hypovolemia 生理盐水

3. cannula / ˈkænjʊlə / *n.* a narrow tube for insertion into a bodily cavity, as for draining off fluid, introducing medication, etc. 插管；套管

4. sterile / ˈsteraɪl / *adj.* free of or using methods to keep free of pathological microorganisms 无菌的

5. electrolytic / ɪˌlektrəˈlɪtɪk / *adj.* of, relating to, or containing an electrolyte 电解质的

6. imbalance / ˌɪmˈbæləns / *n.* a lack of balance or state of disequilibrium 不平衡

7. overload / əʊvəˈləʊd / *v.* to put too many things or people on or into something 使超载；使负荷过重

8. nosocomial / ˌnɒsəˈkəʊmiəl / *adj.* resulting from treatment in a hospital but not related to the original disease, also called *hospital-acquired* 医院的

9. phlebitis / fləˈbaɪtɪs / *n.* inflammation of a vein 静脉炎

10. infiltration / ˌɪnfɪlˈtreɪʃn / *n.* fluid accumulation in the tissues in excess amounts 浸润

11. staphylococcus / ˌstæfɪləˈkɒkəs / *n.* (pl. staphylococci) a group of bacteria which cause local infections and other serious infections 葡萄球菌

12. erythema / ˌerɪˈθiːmə / *n.* redness of the skin caused by injury or infection 红斑

13. tenderness / ˈtendənəs / *n.* a pain that is felt when the area is touched 压痛

14. aseptic / ˌeɪˈseptɪk / *adj.* free of or using methods to keep free of pathological microorganisms 无菌的

15. contamination / kənˌtæmɪˈneɪʃn / *n.* the state of being contaminated 弄脏；污染

16. positional / pəˈzɪʃənəl / *adj.* of or relating to or determined by position 位置的；地位的

17. additive / ˈædətɪv / *n.* any substance which is added to another substance to improve it or prevent deterioration 添加剂

18. dextrose / ˈdekstrəʊz / *n.* an isomer of glucose that is found in honey and sweet fruits 葡萄糖

19. resite / rɪˈzaɪt / *v.* choose another site for... 给……选择新址

20. dehydrated / ˌdiːhaɪˈdreɪtɪd / *adj.* suffering from excessive loss of water from the body 脱水的

21. nuisance / ˈnjuːsns / *n.* a person, thing, or situation that annoys you or causes problems 讨厌（麻烦）的人（事物，情况）

22. KVO: keep vein open / kiːp veɪn ˈəʊpən / fluid is given at a very slow rate via an IV infusion so that the IV line can continue to be used for IV injections or infusions 保持静脉通畅

23. expire / ɪkˈspaɪə(r) / *v.* lose validity 到期，过期，失效

24. expiry / ɪkˈspaɪəri / *n.* coming to an end of a contract period 满期，逾期

25. initial / ɪˈnɪʃl / *adj.* occurring at the beginning 最初的

26. PICC: Peripherally Inserted Central Catheter 外周中心静脉导管

Performing Hygienic Care

Intended Learning Objectives

On completion of the unit, students should be able to:

1. describe the basic objects (items) for personal hygienic care;
2. communicate with patients when tending to morning and evening care;
3. talk about the care of pressure ulcers (bed sores).

Lead-in

Listen and repeat.

Listen to the following sentences and repeat them. Pay attention to the pronunciation and intonation.

1. Would you like some help to wash?
2. I can help you to wash now, if you're ready.
3. Would you like me to give you a hand to shave?
4. Could you please change my sheets? I'm sorry but I've wetted the bed.
5. Would you please make beds from five to ten?
6. Would you prefer a shower or a bed sponge?
7. I'll just get the commode chair and then I can take you down to the bathroom.
8. Could you please tend David White's mouth and eye?
9. I'm just going to clean your mouth with these swabs which have been dipped in mouthwash, OK?
10. I'm just going to use cotton buds soaked with saline to clean the lower part of your nostrils out. We won't go in too far.

Communication Focus
A patient's confidentiality and privacy are of great importance.

In pairs, discuss the following questions.

1. Whom can you communicate with to talk about your patient's treatment or condition?
2. When dealing with patients, what privacy considerations should you be mindful of?

Part One Describing Hygiene Equipment and Giving Hygiene Report

Task 1 Work in pairs. 🎧

Label the pictures with the words in the box, and listen and check. Then describe the function of each object.

Example: *Shaving cream is used to …*

Towel is used to …

gloves	wash basin	towel	toothpaste	toothbrush	soap
swab	shaving cream	shampoo	razor	pyjamas	sink
bin	kidney basin	brush	detergent	blanket	bucket
clinical disposable bag		paper towels			

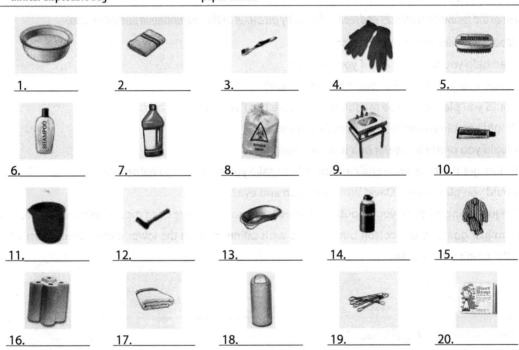

1. _____ 2. _____ 3. _____ 4. _____ 5. _____

6. _____ 7. _____ 8. _____ 9. _____ 10. _____

11. _____ 12. _____ 13. _____ 14. _____ 15. _____

16. _____ 17. _____ 18. _____ 19. _____ 20. _____

Task 2 Pronounce the words. 🎧

Write down the words according to the phonetic symbols below. And then listen and check.

1. / ɪnˈspekʃn / _____
2. / ˈhaɪdʒiːn / _____
3. / ˈspɪlɪdʒ / _____
4. / ˈfluːɪd / _____
5. / ˈjʊərɪn / _____
6. / stɑːf / _____
7. / kənˈsɪdərət / _____
8. / swɒb / _____
9. / spʌndʒ / _____
10. / ˈmaʊθwɒʃ / _____

Task 3 Listen and complete. 🎧

Listen to a short dialogue between a hospital administrator and a ward cleaner. Complete the hygiene report below by filling in the missing words.

Hygiene Report	
Score of ward	1. _____ out of _____
Door handle	2. not _____
Bed	3. not always cleaned _____
Toilet	4. must be cleaned _____ a day but they are only cleaned _____ a day
Floor	5. must be cleaned _____ a day but they are only cleaned _____
Spillages of Bodily Fluid	6. The report says that _____ was 30 minutes to clean up a spill of urine
Washing hand	7. Nurses must wash hands _____
Reason why they didn't do well enough	8. They are really very _____

Note: MRSA, Methicillin-resistant staphylococcus aureus, is a bacterium that causes infections in different parts of the body.

Part Two　Performing Morning Care and Evening Care

Task 4 Listen and complete. 🎧

Listen to a lecture about personal hygiene care and take notes by answering the following questions and completing the sentences. Then practice the dialogue in pairs.

A: What's the purpose of bathing?

B: The primary purpose of bathing is to 1. _____.

A: How many types of baths do you know?

B: 2. _____.

A: What are they?

B: They are 3. _____.

A: How is perineal care done?

B: Well, perineal care is usually done 4. _____ and it is done _____ for patients affected with incontinence and diaphoresis.

A: As for shaving, how often and how do male patients and female patients want?

B: Male patients often want a facial shave 5. _____; female patients usually want _____ shaved about once a week.

A: What does oral hygiene consist of?

B: Well, oral hygiene usually consists of 6. _____. Partial and full _____ are also brushed and rinsed.

A: As for diabetics, how is foot care done?

B: Well, as for diabetics, the feet must be completely cleaned and dried and examined daily for any sign of 7._____.

A: What about patient's hair care?

B: Emm, patient's hair can be washed 8._____ in the shower, bathtub and in bed with a special bed tray or dry shampoo.

A: What should nurses encourage patients to do?

B: Patients should be encouraged to 9._____.

A: Why should the patients' nails appear clean?

B: Because dirt can cause 10._____, and jagged nails may cause _____ to the patients or to the staff attending to them.

Task 5 Work in pairs. 🎧

Listen to the dialogue between a patient and a nurse about the morning care. Answer the related questions and then practice in pairs.

1. Did the patient sleep well last night?

2. What's the matter with his mouth?

3. What is the purpose of stimulating the patient's blood circulation?

4. Why does the patient want to change his clothes?

5. Does the patient need to get out of bed while the nurse is doing the complete change?

Task 6 Work in pairs. 🎧

Listen to a recording and complete the table below. Discuss in pairs what a nurse usually does when tending to morning and evening care.

Morning and Evening Care	
Morning care	Morning care usually includes toileting, 1._____, bathing, 2._____, skin care measures, hair care, dressing, and positioning for comfort and so on.
Self-care patient	In spite of their being able to manage their 3._____ all by themselves, these patients should still be offered a back massage.
Partial care patient	These patients always receive morning hygiene care 4._____ or 5._____ in the bathroom. Because of weakness, these patients can wash only 6._____ that are within easy reach.
Complete care patient	These patients usually need a 7._____ or a bath in the shower or tub.
Evening care	Evening care usually includes 8._____ routinely, changing 9._____, 10._____ comfortably.

Part Three Caring for Pressure Ulcers

Task 7 **Work in pairs.** 🎧

Particular attention should be paid to the areas of bony prominences which are at a high risk for pressure ulcers. Listen and write down the Chinese meaning of each word according to the picture below.

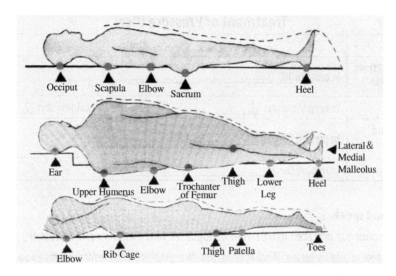

1. occiput _____
2. scapula _____
3. elbow _____
4. sacrum _____
5. heel _____
6. toes _____
7. thigh _____
8. trochanter femur _____
9. lower leg _____
10. upper humerus _____
11. rib cage _____
12. patella_____

Task 8 **Listen and complete.** 🎧

Listen to the following recordings on prevention and treatment of pressure ulcers and complete the table by filling in the missing words. Then discuss in pairs.

Prevention of Pressure Ulcer		
	Patient	**Frequency**
Position change	those who use wheelchairs	change positions every 1._____
	those who spend most of their time in bed	change positions at least 2._____
Daily skin care	check the skin daily for redness or signs of 3._____	
		Reason
	keep the skin moist	If the skin is either too dry or too moist, the damage is 4._____
	never massage bony areas	The skin is too 5._____

Prevention of Pressure Ulcer

Diet and lifestyle change	eat a 6._____ diet
	use good 7._____
	maintain 8._____ levels
	Make sure he/she 9._____

Treatment of Pressure Ulcer

Way	Aim
Using special mattress and bed	in order to 10._____
Dressing	to keep the ulcers 11._____ and the surrounding skin 12._____
Applying drug and chemical	to prevent 13._____
Surgery	to remove the 14._____

Task 9 **Listen and speak.** 🎧

Listen to a sample dialogue and then make a new dialogue on your own. Pay attention to the pronunciation and intonation while listening and imitating. Work in pairs, practice speaking and performing the dialogue.

(Liu Feng learns to provide routine hygienic care for an unconscious patient in the ICU.)

Nurse: Liu Feng, you're welcome to practise here. Now let's go to see Mrs. Brown.

Liu Feng: OK. It seems she's unconscious.

Nurse: Yeah. She is.

Liu Feng: I was taught that the care of an unconscious patient would be a comprehensive one and almost cover all the basic nursing skills.

Nurse: You're quite right. Today we'll just focus on the hygienic care for the patient.

Liu Feng: Personal hygiene usually includes skin care, bathing and the care of mouth, eyes, ears and nose.

Nurse: You get the point. We do oral hygiene twice a day. We use a cotton stick to brush the patient's teeth and mucous membranes, especially the lips. They're easy to get dry and have debris because the unconscious patient often uses the mouth to breathe.

Liu Feng: How do you care for the eyes, ears or nose?

Nurse: Use eye drops, eye ointment, or eye patches to prevent infections. This patient has tubes in her nostrils, so it is essential to lubricate them regularly.

Liu Feng: I see.

Nurse: Skin is the first defence against infections, so we should maintain the patient's skin integrity. Each time after a bed bath, we should dry the patient thoroughly and massage her.

Liu Feng: It can stimulate the blood circulation and prevent bedsores.

Nurse: Right. Do you know what places are prone to bedsores?

Liu Feng: Bone prominences, such as occiput, neck, shoulder, elbow, pelvis and heel, etc. They're usually under pressure so that the blood circulation is poor.

Nurse: In addition to massage, we should turn the patient every 2 hours to relieve pressure. Remember to change bed linens whenever they're wet. Do not drag the patient when moving her.

Liu Feng: There're so many things to learn. I'll keep them in mind.

Role-play

Scenario: at the ward in the morning

Task: Student A acts as a nurse and Student B acts as a patient suffering from bedsores. Make a dialogue about bedsores.

Useful sentences patterns:

1. Did you have a good night?

2. Let me help you to clean up and make you comfortable.

3. Please turn over to the other side. I'll rub your back with a hot towel and then massage it with alcohol and talcum powder.

4. It's mainly to stimulate your blood circulation to prevent bedsores.

5. I'll help you to change at once.

6. I'm also going to change the sheets on your bed.

7. I can do the change without your getting out of bed.

8. I'm feeling better now. Thank you so much.

More Practice

Role-play.

Read the following case and play the roles of a nurse and a patient based on the case. In the dialogue, you should complete the tasks below the case.

> **Case Study:** Mrs. White, a 70-year-old woman, is admitted to hospital for pneumonia. Due to her worsening respiratory status she had found it uncomfortable to lay flat so she had been staying in a chair upright around the clock.

Tasks:

1. Find out the reasons for the patient's ulcer.

2. Explain the assessment of the ulcer.

3. Explain the treatment of the ulcer.

New words

1. ulcer / ˈʌlsə(r) / *n.* a circumscribed inflammatory and often suppurating lesion on the skin or an internal mucous surface resulting in necrosis of tissues 溃疡

2. commode / kəˈməʊd / n. a piece of furniture that looks like a chair but has a toilet under the seat 大便坐椅

3. saline / ˈseɪlaɪn / adj. containing salt 盐的；含盐分的

4. confidentiality / ˌkɒnfɪˌdenʃiˈæləti / n. discretion in keeping secret information 秘密；隐私

5. soak / səʊk / v. submerge in a liquid 浸泡；渗透

6. germ / dʒɜːm / n. a small simple structure (as a fertilized egg) from which new tissue can develop into a complete organism 细菌；胚芽；萌芽

7. nonskid / ˈnɒnˈskɪd / adj. designed to reduce or prevent skidding（轮胎等）不滑的

8. perineal / periˈniːəl / adj. of or relating to the perineum 会阴的

9. odour / ˈəʊdə(r) / n. a smell, especially one that is unpleasant 气味

10. diaphoresis / ˌdaɪəfəˈriːsɪs / n. the process of the sweat glands of the skin secreting a salty fluid 发汗

11. deodorant / diˈəʊdərənt / n. a toiletry applied to the skin in order to mask unpleasant odours 除臭剂

12. anticoagulant / ˌæntikəʊˈæɡjələnt / n. a medicine that prevents or retards the clotting of blood 抗凝剂

13. bleeding / ˈbliːdɪŋ / n. flow of blood from ruptured blood vessels 出血

14. jagged / ˈdʒæɡɪd / adj. having a sharply uneven surface or outline 锯齿状的；参差不齐的

15. tangled / ˈtæŋɡld / adj. in a confused mass 缠结的；纠缠的；紊乱的；复杂的

16. circulation / ˌsɜːkjəˈleɪʃn / n. movement through a circuit; especially the movement of blood through the heart and blood vessels 循环

17. stimulate / ˈstɪmjuleɪt / vt. cause to do; cause to act in a specified manner 刺激

18. underarm / ˈʌndərɑːm / adj. with hand brought forward and up from below shoulder level 腋下的

19. prominence / ˈprɒmɪnəns / n. something that bulges out or is protuberant or projects from a form 突出物

20. occiput / ˈɒksɪpʌt / n. back part of the head or skull 枕骨部；后头部

21. scapula / ˈskæpjʊlə / n. either of two flat triangular bones with one on each side of the shoulder in human beings 肩胛；肩胛骨（复数 scapulas 或 scapulae）

22. sacrum / ˈseɪkrəm/ n. the wedge-shaped bone consisting of five fused vertebrae forming the posterior part of the pelvis; its base connects with the lowest lumbar vertebra and its tip with the coccyx 骶骨；荐骨（复数 sacrums 或 sacra）

23. thigh / θaɪ / n. the part of the leg between the hip and the knee 大腿；股

24. femur / ˈfiːmə(r) / n. the longest and thickest bone of the human skeleton which extends from the pelvis to the knee 股骨；大腿骨（复数 femurs 或 femora）

25. humerus / ˈhjuːmərəs / n. the large bone extending from the shoulder to the elbow 肱部；肱上膊（复数 humeri）

26. patella / pəˈtelə / n. the small flat triangular bone in front of the knee that protects the knee joint 膝盖骨（复数 patellas 或 patellae）

27. spine / spaɪn / n. the series of vertebrae forming the axis of the skeleton and protecting the spinal cord 脊柱；脊椎

28. buttock / ˈbʌtək / n. either of the two large fleshy masses of muscular tissue that form the human rump 半边臀部

29. drainage / ˈdreɪnɪdʒ / n. the process by which water or liquid waste is drained from an area 引流；排水

30. floss / flɒs / n. a soft thread for cleaning the spaces between the teeth 牙线

31. denture / ˈdentʃə(r) / n. a dental appliance that artificially replaces the missing teeth 一副义齿；托牙

32. partial / ˈpɑːʃl / adj. being or affecting only a part; not total 局部的

33. independently / ˌɪndɪˈpendəntli / adv. on your own; without outside help 独立地；自立地

34. secretion / sɪˈkriːʃn / n. a liquid substance produced by parts of the body or plant 分泌物

35. linen / ˈlɪnɪn / n. sheets, pillowcases, etc. made of cloth that are used in the home 亚麻织品

36. assessment / əˈsesmənt / n. the act of judging or assessing a person or situation or event 评定；估价

37. documentation / ˌdɒkjumenˈteɪʃn / n. documentary validation 文件证明

38. spongy / ˈspʌndʒi / adj. like a sponge in being able to absorb liquids and yield it back when compressed 海绵状的；有吸水性的

39. inflamed / ɪnˈfleɪmd / adj. resulting from inflammation; hot and swollen and reddened 发炎的；红肿的

40. serum / ˈsɪərəm / n. watery fluid of the blood that resembles plasma but contains fibrinogen 血清；浆液

41. blister / ˈblɪstə(r) / n. an elevation of the skin filled with serous fluid 水泡；水疱

42. swollen / ˈswəʊlən / adj. abnormally distended especially by fluids or gas 肿胀的；水肿的

43. palpable / ˈpælpəbl / adj. capable of being perceived by the senses or the mind; especially capable of being handled or touched or felt 摸得出的；明显的；可感知的

44. discoloration / ˌdɪsˌkʌləˈreɪʃn / n. a soiled or discolored appearance 变色；污点

45. mattress / ˈmætrəs / n. the soft part of a bed, that you lie on 床垫；底垫

46. moist / mɔɪst / adj. slightly wet 潮湿的

47. unconscious / ʌnˈkɒnʃəs / adj. not conscious; lacking awareness and the capacity for sensory perception as if being asleep or dead 无意识的；失去知觉的；不省人事的

48. hygienic / haɪˈdʒiːnɪk / adj. tending to promote or preserve health 卫生的；保健的

49. mucous / ˈmjuːkəs / adj. of or secreting or covered with or resembling mucus 黏的；分泌黏液的

50. membrane / ˈmembreɪn / n. a thin layer of skin or tissue that connects or covers the parts inside the body 细胞膜；薄膜；膜皮

51. debris / ˈdeɪbriː / n. the remains of something that have been destroyed or broken up 碎片；残骸

52. lubricate / ˈluːbrɪkeɪt / vt. make slippery or smooth through the application of a lubricant 使……润滑；给……加润滑油

53. nostril / ˈnɒstrəl / n. either one of the two external openings to the nasal cavity in the nose 鼻孔

54. pelvis / ˈpelvɪs / n. the structure of the vertebrate skeleton supporting the lower limbs in humans and the hind limbs or corresponding parts in other vertebrates 骨盆（复数 pelvises 或 pelves）

Talking About Nutrition

Intended Learning Objectives

On completion of the unit, students should be able to:

1. describe some essential kinds of nutrients we need;
2. describe the definition of obesity and instruct patients with obesity on nutrition;
3. describe the types of diabetes and instruct patients with diabetes on nutrition.

Lead-in

Listen and repeat. 🎧

Listen to the following sentences and repeat them. Pay attention to the pronunciation and intonation.

1. How has your appetite been lately?
2. Do you feel sick or uncomfortable in any way?
3. I can really understand that you don't feel too hungry with all your discomfort at present, but your body needs the nutrition so that you can regain your strength and energy.
4. Please let us know if there is something you particularly feel like eating.
5. How much food do you normally eat in a day?
6. How big would each meal be?
7. Have you noticed experiencing any weight gain or weight loss lately?
8. The patient is a healthy weight/slightly underweight/obese for her height.
9. How would you describe your diet?
10. What kinds of food does your diet mostly consist of ?

Communication Focus

Open-ended questions will generally lead to more detailed and expressive answers.

In pairs, discuss the following questions.

1. What are open-ended questions?
2. Why should we use more open-ended questions?
3. Compare the following questions used when taking patient's history and express your opinion.

Open-ended: Do you have a history of any medical problems?

Closed: Do you have a history of heart disease? / Do you have a history of respiratory illness? / Do you have a history of diabetes? / Have you had any operations before?

Part One   Describing Nutrition

Task 1 **Work in pairs.**

Look at the following menu and discuss with your partner based on the table below.

Main Course A	Main Course B	Dessert
two grilled burgers	fried rice	chocolate pudding
tuna fish pie	boiled potatoes	a banana
a cheese pizza	salad	a doughnut
lentil soup	baked beans in tomato sauce	yoghurt
egg noodles	tinned tomatoes	**Drink**
two slices of roast beef	stir-fried mushrooms	a bottle of cola
two fried eggs	fried onion rings	a glass of orange juice
tofu curry	steamed broccoli	a glass of wine
a lamb kebab		a glass of milk

Category	Food Item
Good source of protein	
Good source of carbohydrate	
Dairy product	
High in fat	
High in vitamin C	
Low in vitamin	
Junk food	
High in calory	
Way of cooking food	

Task 2 **Pronounce the words.** 🎧

Write down the words according to the phonetic symbols below. And then listen and check.

1. / ˈʃʊgə(r) / _____
2. / ˈprəʊtiːn / _____
3. / ˈdeəri / _____
4. / fæts / _____
5. / helθ / _____
6. / ˈvɪtəmɪn / _____
7. / ˈmɪnərəl / _____
8. / ˈenədʒi / _____
9. / ˈkælsiəm / _____
10. / ˌkɑːbəʊˈhaɪdreɪt / _____

Read and complete.

Look at the food group table. Complete the blanks in Column 2 with the words in the box. And then share the information with your partner.

fight	repair	fuel	digest
bones	energy	blood	skin

Food group	What do they do for your body?	Where can you find them?
carbohydrate	They provide a great part of the 1._____ in our diets.	potatoes, rice, bread
fat	They are stored in the body for later use when carbohydrates are in short supply. They 2._____ the body and help absorb some vitamins.	meat, oils, sweets, dairy products
mineral	Calcium is good for your 3._____. Iron is good for the 4._____. Zinc helps you 5._____ against infection.	fresh fruits and vegetables (zinc in seafood)
protein	They build up, maintain, and 6._____ the tissues in your body.	meat, fish, beans, eggs, dairy products
vitamin A / B / C / D / E	They are essential for your 7._____, bones and teeth.	fresh fruits and vegetables, dairy products
fibre	It helps you to 8._____ your food.	fresh fruits, corn, beans, whole grains

Part Two　Helping Patient with Obesity

Task 4 **Listen and complete.** 🎧

Listen to the dialogue and complete the Nursing Assessment Form and the following sentences. And then practice the dialogue with your partner.

Diet restrictions and requirements	( ) yes ( ) no	If YES _____ _____ _____
a. BMI _____		
b. Food allergies	( ) yes ( ) no	If YES _____ _____
c. Last meal (date / time) _____	Give details _____ _____	

Tick the correct information based on the dialogue.

1. The patient's BMI indicates he is (slightly overweight / slightly underweight).

2. The patient wants to (gain weight / lose weight).

3. The patient's (current weight / normal weight) is sixty-six kilos.

4. The patient (overeats / doesn't eat enough).

Note:

BMI (body mass index) is used to decide if a person's weight is healthy or not. To calculate a person's
BMI, we use the formula: (weight in kilograms) / (height in metres)^2

Readings: BMI of less than 18. 5 is underweight.

BMI from 18. 5 to 24. 9 is the right weight for women.

BMI from 20. 5 to 25. 0 is the right weight for men.

BMI of 25.0 to 29. 9 is overweight.

BMI of more than 30 is obese.

Task 5 **Work in pairs.** 🎧

Put these words in order to make sentences. Listen and check your answer.

1. kind, diet, for, do, of, you, What, me, recommend?

2. it, patients, five, a, day, six, or, Some, find, eat, meals, helpful, to, small, times.

3. has, lately, How, appetite, been, your?

4. needs, body, you, Your, can, strength, energy, your, regain, nutrition, so, that, and, the.

5. associated, increased, Excess, heart, of, an, disease, is, with, risk, weight.

6. should, You, avoid, fried, to, in, order, fatty, blood, high, prevent, meat, foods, cholesterol, and.

Task 6 **Role-play.** 🎧

Listen to the recording and play the role.

Scenario: in the admitting room

Instruments needed: a body mass index calculator, a weight scale, a height measuring gauge and a chart

Task: Student A plays as a nurse to measure height and weight for student B who plays as a patient.
And swap the role later.

Information for Student B:

Height	Weight
5ft 6in	211 lb

Useful sentence patterns:

1. Would you mind telling me what your weight is / how much you weigh?

2. Your height, please? / How tall are you?

3. How severe is my weight problem?

4. A patient with a body mass index of 25 to 29. 9 is considered overweight.

5. Without intervention, what should I expect?

6. How much weight should I lose?

7. A weight loss goal should be realistic.

8. What kind of diet do you recommend for me?

9. Does meal frequency matter?

10. Some patients find it helpful to eat small meals five or six times a day.

Part Three　Helping Patient with Diabetes

Task 7 **Listen and complete.** 🎧

Complete the passage according to the recording, and then repeat it.

What is Diabetes?

Diabetes is a disease that occurs when your blood 1.＿＿＿＿＿＿ , also called blood sugar, is too high. Blood glucose is your main source of energy and comes from the food you eat. Insulin, a 2.＿＿＿＿＿＿ made by the pancreas, helps glucose from food get into your cells to be used for energy. Sometimes your body doesn't make enough—or any—insulin or doesn't use insulin well. Glucose then stays in your blood and doesn't reach your cells.

Over time, having too much glucose in your blood can cause health problems. Although diabetes has no 3.＿＿＿＿＿＿ , you can take steps to manage your diabetes and stay healthy.

Sometimes people call diabetes "a touch of sugar" or " 4.＿＿＿＿＿＿ diabetes". These terms suggest that someone doesn't really have diabetes or has a less serious case, but every case of diabetes is serious.

The most common types of diabetes are type 1, type 2, and 5.＿＿＿＿＿＿ diabetes.

Task 8 **Listen and choose the best answer.** 🎧

Listen to the recording and then choose the best answer to each question.

1. What's wrong with the patient? He has (a)＿＿＿＿＿＿.

    a. headache   b. flu   c. fever   d. nausea

2. Does he feel tired and itchy?＿＿＿＿＿＿.

    a. Yes   b. No   c. He has no idea   d. Not mentioned

3. How is his appetite?＿＿＿＿＿＿.

    a. Very good   b. Bad   c. Common   d. Not sure

4. How long did the symptoms last?＿＿＿＿＿＿.

    a. Less than six months   b. More than six months

    c. More than three months   d. More than four months

5. What will the nurse do?＿＿＿＿＿＿.

    a. She will take an X-ray picture of his stomach and intestine

    b. She will ask the patient to come to the hospital for treatment

    c. She will give the patients 2 tablets twice a day, morning and evening

    d. She will take his urine and blood samples to check their sugar contents

Task 9 **Complete and practice.** 🎧

Fill in the blanks and then listen and check the answers. Act it out in pairs with your partner.

(After the consultation)

P: Dr. Wang told me I have diabetes.

N: Yes, I know. 1._____?

P: Yes, my father has it.

N: Dr. Wang has ordered that you should follow a 2._____ diet and 3._____.
Here are instructions for your therapy, which by the way, you'll have to administer by yourself at home. We'll help you if you find it difficult. Here are some medicines for your headache.

P: Thank you very much. 4._____?

N: As the doctor told you, you should stick to a special diet and avoid 5._____.

P: 6._____?

N: You'd better learn something about diabetes and have your 7._____ tested regularly.
Please stick to your new diet, take your medicine regularly and 8._____. I'm sure you will feel better soon.

P: Thank you for your advice.

More Practice

Role-play.

Read the following case and play the roles of a nurse and a patient based on the case. In the dialogue, you should complete the tasks below the case.

Case Study: Mr. Black is in his mid-thirties, and in an intensive exercise program. He is currently underweight and would like to gain weight healthily while continuing to exercise. He wants advice on a suitable diet.

Tasks:

1. Explain about eating a balanced diet.

2. Suggest additional carbohydrate and lean protein food.

3. Emphasize the need to avoid fatty meat and fried foods in order to prevent high blood cholesterol.

4. Recommend other ways for him to gain weight safely.

New words

1. nutrition / njuˈtrɪʃn / *n.* the organic process of nourishing or being nourished; the process by which an organism assimilates food and uses it for growth and maintenance 营养

2. essential / ɪˈsenʃl / *adj.* basic and fundamental 基本的；必要的；本质的

3. nutrient / 'nju:triənt / n. any substance that can be metabolized by an organism to give energy and build 营养物；滋养物

4. instruct / ɪn'strʌkt / vt. impart skills or knowledge to 指导

5. obesity / əʊ'bi:səti / n. more than average fatness 肥大；肥胖

6. appetite / 'æpɪtaɪt / n. a feeling of craving food etc. 食欲；嗜好

7. uncomfortable / ʌn'kʌmftəbl / adj. conducive to or feeling mental discomfort 不舒服的；不安的

8. discomfort / dɪs'kʌmfət / n. the state of being tense and feeling pain 不适；不安

9. obese / əʊ'bi:s / adj. excessively fat 肥胖的；过胖的

10. grilled / grɪld / adj. cooked by radiant heat (as over a grill) 烤的

11. tuna / 'tju:nə / n. a large sea fish caught for food 金枪鱼；鲔鱼

12. lentil / 'lentl / n. a round flat seed like a bean used for food 兵豆；小扁豆

13. tofu / 'təʊfu: / n. cheeselike food made of curdled soybean milk 豆腐

14. lamb / læm / n. the flesh of a young domestic sheep eaten as food 羔羊肉

15. kebab / kɪ'bæb / n. small pieces of meat and vegetables cooked on a stick 烤肉串（等于 kabob）

16. tinned / tɪnd / adj. sealed in a can or jar 罐头的；听装的

17. steamed / sti:md / adj. cooked in steam 蒸熟的；蒸的

18. broccoli / 'brɒkəli / n. a plant with dense clusters of tight green flower buds 花椰菜；西兰花

19. doughnut / 'dəʊnʌt / n. a small round cake, often in the form of a ring 油炸圈饼

20. yogurt / 'jɒgət / n. a custard-like food made from curdled milk 酸奶；酸乳酪

21. figure / 'fɪgə(r) / n. an alternative name for the body of a human being（人的）体形

22. dairy / 'deəri / adj. made from milk 牛奶的；乳品的

23. fat / fæt / n. a solid or liquid substance from animals or plants, treated so that it becomes pure for use in cooking（食用的）动植物油

24. vitamin / 'vɪtəmɪn / n. any of a group of organic substances essential in small quantities to normal metabolism 维生素

25. mineral / 'mɪnərəl / n. a substance that is formed naturally in the earth, such as coal, salt, stone, or gold 矿物；无机物

26. calcium / 'kælsiəm / n. a white metallic element that helps to form teeth, bones, and chalk 钙

27. carbohydrate / kɑ:bəʊ'haɪdreɪt / n. an essential structural component of living cells and source of energy for animals; it includes simple sugar with small molecules as well as macromolecular substances 碳水化合物；糖类

28. fibre / 'faɪbə(r) / n. the part of food that helps to keep a person healthy by keeping the bowels working and moving other food quickly through the body 纤维素

29. zinc / zɪŋk / n. a mineral which is neccessary for human health. Zinc deficiency can cause reduced ability to taste food and other problems 锌

30. digest / daɪ'dʒest / vt. convert food into absorbable substances 消化；吸收

31. BMI: body mass index 身体质量指数；体质指数

32. allergic / ə'lɜ:dʒɪk / adj. characterized by or caused by allergy 对……过敏的；对……极讨厌的

33. peanut / ˈpiːnʌt / n. a nut that grows underground in a thin shell 花生

34. lactose / ˈlæktəʊs / n. a type of sugar found in milk and used in some baby foods 乳糖

35. intolerance / ɪnˈtɒlərəns / n. an inability to take particular medicine or eat particular foods without suffering bad effects 不耐受

36. toast / təʊst / n. slices of bread that have been heated 烤面包；吐司

37. administer / ədˈmɪnɪstə(r) / vt. work in an administrative capacity; supervise 管理；执行

38. overweight / ˌəʊvəˈweɪt / n. the property of excessive fatness 超重

39. intervention / ˌɪntəˈvenʃn / n. the act of intervening (as to mediate a dispute) 介入；干预

40. stroke / strəʊk / n. a sudden loss of consciousness resulting when the rupture or occlusion of a blood vessel leads to oxygen lack in the brain 中风

41. gallstone / ˈɡɔːlstəʊn / n. a hard painful means that can form in the gall bladder 胆结石

42. permanent / ˈpɜːmənənt / adj. continuing or enduring without marked change in status or condition or place 永久的；永恒的；不变的

43. realistic / ˌriːəˈlɪstɪk / adj. aware or expressing awareness of things as they really are 现实的

44. category / ˈkætəɡəri / n. a collection of things sharing a common attribute 种类；分类

45. regimen / ˈredʒɪmən / n. a set of rules about food and exercise that some people follow in order to stay healthy 生活规则；养生法；养生之道

46. macronutrient / ˌmaɪkrəʊˈnjuːtriənt / n. a substance needed only in small amounts for normal body function (e. g. vitamins or minerals) 主要营养素

47. glucose / ˈɡluːkəʊs / n. a monosaccharide sugar that has several forms; an important source of physiological energy 葡萄糖

48. insulin / ˈɪnsjəlɪn / n. a chemical substance produced in the body that controls the amount of sugar in the blood 胰岛素

49. hormone / ˈhɔːməʊn / n. a chemical substance produced in the body or in plant that encourages growth or influences how the cells and tissues fuction 激素；荷尔蒙

50. pancreas / ˈpæŋkriəs / n. a large elongated exocrine gland located behind the stomach which secretes pancreatic juice and insulin 胰腺

51. borderline / ˈbɔːdəlaɪn / adj. of questionable or minimal quality 边界的

52. gestational / dʒeˈsteɪʃənəl / adj. of or relating to gestation 妊娠期的；受孕的

53. subside / səbˈsaɪd / vi. wear off or die down 平息；减弱

54. itchy / ˈɪtʃi / adj. causing an irritating cutaneous sensation 发痒的

55. therapy / ˈθerəpi / n. the act of caring for someone (as by medication or remedial training etc.) 治疗；疗法（复数 therapies）

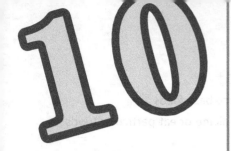

Caring for Pre-Operative Patients

Intended Learning Objectives

On completion of the unit, students should be able to:

1. do pre-operative assessment;
2. prepare patients for surgery;
3. use pre-operative checklists.

Lead-in

Listen and repeat. 🎧

Listen to the following sentences and repeat them. Pay attention to the pronunciation and intonation.

1. We are going to do the operation on you tomorrow.
2. I'm afraid you'll have to be operated on for appendicitis.
3. We'll give you anaesthesia.
4. If you feel any pain during the operation, just let me know.
5. Have you signed the consent yet?
6. I'd like to shave off the hair around the operation area.
7. I'll give you an enema tonight.
8. After that, please don't take any food or water before the operation.
9. The purpose of this is to make sure that you have an empty stomach when you have surgery.
10. Please remove all nail polish, gel or similar nails on the both hands prior to the time of surgery.

Communication Focus

The patient's emotions and grief are important and need to be acknowledged and accepted: show empathy.

In pairs, discuss the following questions.

1. Can you list some basic rules that you can use to deal with the patient's emotions?
2. What strategies can you use to relieve the patient's anxiety before or after the surgery?
3. What strategies may be effective for a pre-op child?

Part One   Doing Pre-Operative Checks

Task 1 **Pronounce the words.** 🎧

Write down the words according to the phonetic symbols below. And then listen and check.

1. / ˌɒpəˈreɪʃn / _____

2. / ˈsɪɡnətʃə(r) / _____

3. / əˈniːsθətɪst / _____

4. / ˌæntiˈseptɪk / _____

5. / ˌɪntəˈfɪə(r) / _____

6. / ˈfluːɪd / _____

7. / ˈmʌsl / _____

8. / ˈenəmə / _____

Task 2 **Listen and complete.** 🎧

Marie Wiseman, 45-year-old, is admitted for chronic appendicitis and ready for appendectomy. Nancy, the Ward Nurse, prepares Mrs. Wiseman for her operation by telling her about the pre-operative routine. Listen to the conversation and complete the following sentences.

1. Yes. _____ _____ _____ look at the operation list when it comes out later today so I can tell you where you are on the list.

2. Now, _____ get you to take off your nail polish later today so the anaesthetist will be able to see your nail beds.

3. And _____ also need to shower with this antiseptic wash.

4. _____ my tummy be shaved before the operation?

5. _____ _____ _____ order you clear fluids for today.

6. Does that mean I _____ be able to eat or drink anything after midnight, _____ I?

7. No, not at all. _____ get you to take a special bowel preparation drink later to clean out your bowel. _____ also need a small enema to help you to open your bowels.

Task 3 **Work in pairs.** 🎧

Listen again and discuss the following questions. And then act out this dialogue.

1. What pre-op hygiene instructions does the nurse give Mrs. Wiseman?

2. Why isn't she allowed to eat or drink before the operation?

3. Why does she have to wear the stockings?

Part Two   Preparing Patient for Surgery

Task 4 **Read and match.**

Match the medical terms (1-6) to their meanings (a-f). And introduce the terms to your partner.

1. indwelling catheter	a. as a little incision into the body as possible, through the use of techniques such as keyhole surgery and laser treatment
2. minimally invasive	b. an abnormal mass of tissue that serves no purpose
3. anaesthetic	c. a tube which is inserted in the bladder to pass urine
4. tumour	d. a medical instrument which is inserted into the abdomen to view the stomach
5. apprehensive	e. drug which blocks pain and other sensations and is used before an operation is performed
6. gastroscope	f. worried or nervous about something that you are going to do

Task 5 Listen and answer. 🎧

Mr. Kim, 50-year-old, is booked for tumour resection under gastroscope tomorrow. Listen to Nadia, the Ward Nurse, explaining what Mr. Kim can expect when he returns to the ward after his operation, and answer the following questions.

1. How is Mr. Kim feeling about his operation?

2. What kind of surgery is he going to have?

3. What is the name of the instrument the surgeon will use to visualize his stomach?

4. Why won't he have a large scar after his operation?

5. Why will Mr. Kim feel nothing during the surgery?

6. When can he eat and drink after his operation?

7. When will the nurse remove his urinary catheter?

Task 6 Work in pairs.

If you are having an abdominal surgery, how much will the following things worry you? Mark them between 0 (it wouldn't worry me at all) and 5 (it would worry me a lot). Discuss the answers with your partner. Imagine your patient has those worries, comfort him/her.

a. dying during surgery   _____

b. having the wrong operation done   _____

c. infection   _____

d. pain after the operation   _____

e. pain during the operation   _____

f. scarring   _____

Part Three   Using Pre-Operative Checklists

Task 7 Listen and complete. 🎧

Angela, the Ward Nurse, is checking Natasha Slessor for a surgery. Listen to the conversation and complete the form mentioned in the conversation of the Pre-operative Checklist. Tick in the appropriate boxes marked YES or NO or N / A (Not Applicable).

Patient Pre-Operative Checklist	U / N: 2018414 Surname: Slessor Given names: Natasha DOB: 3 / 7 / 1965 Sex: Female

To be used as an added check so that the patient is fully prepared for his/her visit to the Operating Theatre.
1. To be signed by the nursing staff on completion of patient's preparation for the Operating Theatre.
2. To be counter-checked by the nurse receiving the patient in the Operating Theatre.

NB: When the check is completed, tick the appropriate column.	**YES**	**NO or N / A**	**O / T**
1. Identification bracelets correct and correctly worn (x2)			
2. Consent form signed			
3. Operation site marked by surgeon			
4. Chart correct, including Drug Chart, Prescription Chart, Notes, Fluid Charts			
5. X-rays included with Charts and Patient Notes			
6. Any known allergies (Red bracelet worn Yes / No)			
7. Caps, crowns, bridges Identify position			
8. Dentures removed (if not removed on ward, please state)			
9. Operation site shaved			
10. Nail polish removed			
11. Jewellery removed or taped			
12. Identify piercings			
13. Theatre gown worn / anti-embolic stockings / knickers			
14. Pre-med given as per anaesthetic chart			
Urine last voided at _____ a.m. / p.m. Catheterized at a.m. / p.m. or _____ N / A			
Fluid last given at _____ a.m. / p.m. Food last given at _____ a.m. / p.m.			
Prepared by (Nursing staff- Ward) A. Faisal (RN) Date: 4/10/2018 Time 10: 00 a.m. / p.m.			
Received by (Nursing staff-Theatre) J. Symons (RN) Date: 4/10/2018 Time 10: 15 a.m. / p.m.			

Task 8 **Listen and complete.** 🎧

Julia, the Theatre Nurse, checks the patient's details related to the operation. She uses the area in the column marked O / T (Operating Theatre). Listen to the conversation and tick the sections of the Checklist that Julia double-checks.

Task 9 Work in pairs. 🎧

Discuss and put the sentences into correct order and then listen to the conversation again and check your answer. Act the conversation out.

☐ a. Can you tell me your full name, please?

☐ b. I'll sign the Checklist, and you've already got a theatre cap to cover your hair.

☐ c. Is this your signature on the consent form?

☐ d. I know you've already answered many of these questions, but we like to double-check everything.

☐ e. I'm going to check you in today.

☐ f. Can you tell me what operation you're having today?

☐ g. I'm just going to go through this Checklist again.

☐ h. Have you had a pre-med?

☐ i. Did you sign a consent form for the operation?

☐ j. I'll have a quick look at your identification bracelet if I may?

More Practice

Role-play.

Read the following case and play the roles of a nurse and a patient based on the case. In the dialogue, you should complete the tasks below the case.

Case Study: David, a 30-year-old man, has been admitted for an elective appendicectomy. He is very stressed about the operation. You are asked to assist the patient with the pre-operative preparation and the post-operative pain intervention.

Tasks:

1. Reassure the patient about anaesthetic management during the operation.

2. Explain post-operative feelings and how to use the analgesic pump.

New words

1. anxiety / æŋˈzaɪəti / n. the feeling of being very worried about something 焦虑；不安；担心

2. anaesthesia / ænəsˈθiːziə / n. loss of bodily sensation with or without loss of consciousness 麻醉；麻木

3. consent / kənˈsent / n. the permission to do something 同意；许可

4. enema / ˈenəmə / n. a liquid that is put into someone's rectum to make their bowels empty 灌肠剂

5. nail polish / ˈneɪl pɒlɪʃ / coloured or transparent liquid which you paint on your nails to make them look attractive 指甲油

6. anaesthetist / əˈniːsθətɪst / n. a doctor or a nurse who has been specially trained to give people

anaesthetics 麻醉师

7. antiseptic / ˌænti'septɪk / adj. helping to prevent infection 抗菌的；抗感染的；消毒的

8. sachet / 'sæʃeɪ / n. a small plastic or paper package containing a liquid or powder 小袋；香包

9. tummy / 'tʌmi / n. stomach—used especially by or to children 肚子；胃

10. interfere / ˌɪntə'fɪə(r) / vi. to deliberately get involved in a situation where you are not wanted or needed 干涉；妨碍；打扰

11. fluid / 'fluːɪd / n. a liquid 液体；流体

12. anaesthetic / ˌænəs'θetɪk / n. a drug that stops you feeling pain 麻醉剂；麻药

13. inhale / ɪn'heɪl / vt. to breathe in air, smoke, or gas 吸入；吸气

14. anti-embolic / 'æntɪ em'bɒlɪk / adj. preventing the formation of embolus 抗栓子的

15. vein / veɪn / n. one of the tubes which carries blood to your heart from other parts of your body 静脉

16. thrombosis / θrɒm'bəʊsɪs / n. a serious medical problem caused by a clot forming in your blood that prevents the blood from flowing normally 血栓形成；血栓症

17. clot / klɒt / n. a thick almost solid mass formed when blood dries 凝块；凝结

18. scar / skɑː(r) / n. a permanent mark that is left on your skin after you have had a cut or wound 伤疤；疤痕

19. minimally invasive / 'mɪnɪməli ɪn'veɪsɪv / involving as little incision into the body as possible, through the use of techniques such as keyhole surgery and laser treatment 微创性的

20. gastroscope / 'gæstrəskəʊp / n. a medical instrument for examining the interior of the stomach 胃镜；胃窥镜

21. incision / ɪn'sɪʒn / n. a neat cut made into something, especially during a medical operation 切口；割口

22. tumour / 'tjuːmə(r) / n. a mass of diseased cells in your body that have divided and increased too quickly 肿瘤；瘤

23. puncture / 'pʌŋktʃə(r) / n. a small hole made by a sharp point, especially in someone's body 穿刺；穿孔

24. drip / drɪp / n. a piece of equipment used in hospitals for putting liquids directly into your blood through a tube 静脉滴注

25. indwelling catheter / ɪn'dwelɪŋ 'kæθɪtə(r) / a thin tube that is put into your body to remove liquids 内置导管

26. pre-med / priː med / n. the drugs administered to sedate patients or otherwise prepare a patient for general anaesthesia 术前用药；麻醉前用药

27. verify / 'verɪfaɪ / vt. to discover whether something is correct or true 核实；核对

28. identity bracelet / aɪ'dentɪti 'breɪslət / a band or chain that you wear around your wrist which contains your personal details 身份腕带

29. ligament / 'lɪgəmənt / n. a band of strong material in your body, similar to muscle, that joins bones or holds an organ in its place 韧带

30. arthroscopy / ɑː'θrɒskrəpɪ / n. the examination of the joint with an arthroscope while making

repairs through a small incision 关节镜检查，关节镜术

31. X-ray / 'eks reɪ / n. a radiogram made by exposing photographic film to X-rays; used in medical diagnosis X 光，X 射线

32. piercing / 'pɪəsɪŋ / n. a hole made through part of your body so that you can put jewellery there, or the process of making these holes 孔，洞眼；（在身体部位）穿孔

33. gown / gaʊn / n. a long loose piece of clothing worn in a hospital by someone doing or having an operation 外科手术服

34. knickers / 'nɪkəz / n. a piece of women's underwear worn between the waist and the top of the legs 灯笼裤；女用短裤

35. bloodstream / 'blʌdstriːm / n. the blood flowing in your body 血流；体内循环的血液

36. overdose / 'əʊvədəʊs / n. too much of a drug taken at one time 用药过量；服药过多

37. IV pump / pʌmp / a piece of medical equipment that can administer fluids via IV 静脉输液泵

Caring for Post-Operative Patients

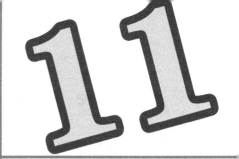

Intended Learning Objectives

On completion of the unit, students should be able to:

1. give a post-operative handover;
2. check a post-operative patient in the ward;
3. give post-operative instructions using appropriate English.

Lead-in

Listen and repeat. 🎧

Listen to the following sentences and repeat them. Pay attention to the pronunciation and intonation.

1. I've got David Smith back from the Theatres.
2. I'll just go through the operation report with you.
3. I'm awake now, but I still feel a bit groggy.
4. I feel as if I want to go to the toilet all the time.
5. That's OK. It takes a little while to be orientated again after an anaesthetic.
6. Patients who've had abdominal surgery are often in quite a bit of discomfort.
7. I know, but this is very helpful for your recovery quickly.
8. Then I'll put up the head of the bed and let the bed do the work of sitting you up.
9. Remember to take deep breaths and look straight ahead—don't look down, are you ready?
10. And try to move further distance next time; you can use the IV pole to hold onto when you are walking.

Communication Focus

A patient's autonomy and independence should be respected and promoted.

In pairs, discuss the following questions.

1. Why is respecting and promoting a patient's autonomy and independence essential?
2. How could you promote a patient's autonomy and independence?

Part One   Giving Post-Operative Handover

Task 1 Pronounce the words. 🎧

Write down the words according to the phonetic symbols below. And then listen and check.

1. / splɪˈnektəmi / _____

2. /ˈθerəpi / _____

3. /ˈpeθədiːn / _____

4. /ˈdekstrəʊz / _____

5. /ˌænəlˈdʒiːziə / _____

6. /ˌkɒmplɪˈkeɪʃn / _____

Task 2 Work in pairs.

Match the abbreviations (1-5) to their meanings (a-e). And try to explain every term to your partner.

(   ) 1. GCS

(   ) 2. neuro obs

(   ) 3. oxygen sats/SaO₂

(   ) 4. NAD

(   ) 5. prn

a. Glasgow Coma Scale; it records the conscious state of a patient

b. Non-Adhesive Dressing

c. measuring of the amount of oxygen which is loaded or saturated into the red blood cells as they pass through the lungs

d. from the Latin *pro re nata*: take whenever required

e. observations which assess neurological functions and include a GCS assessment

Task 3 Listen and complete. 🎧

David Smith, a 36-year-old patient who has had a surgery following a road traffic accident (RTA), comes back to the ward. Mary, the Recovery Nurse, hands David over to Anne, the Ward Nurse. Anne conducts an initial return-to-ward check and starts David on post-op observations. Listen to the conversation and complete the chart below. After that, act it out.

~~RTA~~	NAD	clips	dextrose	intact	oral	redivac	patent
72	75	97	36°C	13/15			

Name of patient	David Smith
Operation performed	Splenectomy post 1. RTA
GCS before leaving Recovery	2. _____
Observation	T 3. _____ P4. _____ BP 112/64 SaO₂ 5. _____ % on 3L/min
IV therapy	1L 5% 6. _____

Name of patient	David Smith
Drain	Redivac × 1, 7._____ and draining small amounts
Wound closure	8._____ ×6
Wound	Covered with 9._____
Analgesia	Pethidine 10._____ mg IM 3° for 3 days then 11._____ analgesia
Post-op instructions	Remove 12._____ when draining <20ml/day Leave dressing 13._____ until surgeon's review

Part Two   Checking Post-Operative Patient in the Ward

Task 4 Pronounce the words. 🎧

Write down the words according to the phonetic symbols below. And then listen and check.

1. / ˌhaɪpəˈθɜːmiə / _____   2. /ˈgrɒgi / _____

3. /ˌænəsˈθetɪk / _____   4. / riˈækʃn / _____

5. / senˈseɪʃn / _____

Task 5 Work in pairs. 🎧

Discuss with your partner what will be the appropriate responses to patients' complaints. Then listen and check the answer. After that, practise how to respond to the complaints.

(   ) 1. I'm still feeling cold. Is that normal?

(   ) 2. I'm awake now, but I still feel a bit groggy.

(   ) 3. My throat feels really sore. It's hard to swallow.

(   ) 4. I feel like I'd be sick if I ate anything.

(   ) 5. I'm in bad pain, and everything hurts.

(   ) 6. I feel like I can't move because it's going to be painful.

(   ) 7. I feel as if I want to go to the toilet all the time.

(   ) 8. I feel dizzy, too. It's like I'm going to fall out of bed.

---

a. That's OK. It takes a little while to be orientated again after an anaesthetic. I'm going to put these bed rails up while you're feeling a bit wobbly and get you some pain relief. Here's the call bell if you need me.

b. That's quite normal. Patients who've had abdominal surgery are often in quite a bit of discomfort. I'll get you an injection for the pain.

c. Yeah, it's OK. It's called hypothermia. It happens sometimes if the operation takes a long time. I'll get you an extra blanket to help warm you up.

d. It's quite common to avoid any movement which might cause discomfort, but it's important that I help you to move around and change positions.

---

e. That's because you've had an anaesthetic. You'll feel better soon.

f. It's quite usual to have that sensation, even though you've got a catheter in your bladder.

g. Nausea is sometimes a reaction to post-operative pain. I'll keep an eye on that.

h. Don't worry, that's normal. It's just caused by the tube they put down your throat during the surgery. I'll get you some ice chips to suck soon.

Task 6 Role-play.

Do a role-play according to Task 5. Student A is a nurse; student B is a post-operative patient.

Part Three   Giving Post-Operative Instructions

Task 7 Listen and complete. 🎧

Listen to the conversation and fill in the blanks with the right words.

1. Your doctor told me that you cannot drink anything right now, because you need to give your _____ a rest.

2. I can help you gargle, but don't drink it, just _____ and _____ it into the emesis basin.

3. Let me help you to get out of bed, maybe you will feel _____ and _____ for the first time.

4. It is necessary to get out of bed right away so you won't get _____ or _____ problems.

5. Put your feet over the _____ and put your arm on my _____. I'll help you sit up.

Task 8 Listen and answer. 🎧

Listen to the conversation again and then answer the following questions.

1. How is the patient feeling after the surgery?

2. Can he stand the pain?

3. What medicines should he have after the surgery?

Task 9 Role-play.

Practise the conversation. Student A is a nurse; Student B is a post-operative patient. Swap roles and practise again.

More Practice

Role-play.

Read the following case and play the roles of a nurse and a patient based on the case. In the dialogue, you should complete the tasks below the case.

Case Study: Ali, a 30-year-old man, has been admitted for multiple injuries in a serious car accident. He has had a surgery for six hours in the operating room. After the surgery, he is in pains. During the morning rounds, the nurse-in-charge, Lily, asks Ali about his pains and gives some instructions to relieve the pains.

Tasks:

1. Find out where the pains are and the severity.

2. Figure out how to control the post-operative pains.

New words

1. splenectomy / splɪˈnektəmi / *n.* the surgical removal of the spleen 脾切除术

2. pethidine /ˈpeθədiːn / *n.* a synthetic opioid pain medication indicated for the treatment of moderate to severe pain 哌替啶（麻醉镇痛药）

3. groggy /ˈgrɒgi / *adj.* stunned or confused and slow to react (as from blows or drunkenness or exhaustion) 酒醉的；无力的

4. GCS: Glasgow Coma Scale a neurological scale which aims to give a reliable and objective way of recording the conscious state of a person 格拉斯哥昏迷指数

5. hypothermia /ˌhaɪpəˈθɜːmiə / *n.* the subnormal body temperature 降低体温；低体温症

6. reaction / riˈækʃn / *n.* a response that reveals a person's feelings or attitude 反应；感应

7. sensation / senˈseɪʃn / *n.* an unelaborated elementary awareness of stimulation 感觉

8. clip / klɪp / *n.* a small metal or plastic object used for holding things together or in place 夹子；回形针

9. NAD: non-addhesive dressing a dressing which doesn't stick to the wound 非黏性敷料

10. orientate /ˈɔːriənteɪt / *v.* determine one's position with reference to another point 确定方向

11. rail / reɪl / *n.* a wooden or metal bar placed around sth. as a barrier or to provide support 栏杆；扶手；围栏

12. gargle /ˈgaːgl / *v.* to wash inside your mouth and throat by moving a liquid around at the back of your throat and then spitting it out 漱口

13. spit / spɪt / *v.* to force liquid, food, etc. out of your mouth 吐；唾

14. emesis /ˈemɪsɪs / *n.* the technical name for vomiting 呕吐

15. constipation / ˌkɒnstɪˈpeɪʃən / *n.* the condition of being unable to get rid of waste materials from the bowels easily 便秘

16. woozy /ˈwuːzi / *adj.* feeling unsteady, confused and unable to think clearly or feeling as if you might vomit 眩晕的；恶心的

Caring for the Elderly

Intended Learning Objectives

On completion of the unit, students should be able to:

1. talk about the physical effects of ageing;
2. assess an elderly care home residents;
3. talk about the physical problems and aids of the elderly;
4. contribute to the healthy development of the elderly.

Lead-in

Listen and repeat. 🎧

Listen to the following sentences and repeat them. Pay attention to the pronunciation and intonation.

1. I'm just going to ask you some questions first so that we can get to know you better. Is that OK?
2. What would you like us to call you?
3. It's your first day here; how do you feel?
4. I understand it's difficult for you at the moment. I hope we can make it easier for you. We're going to try, anyway.
5. Do you have any favorite foods?
6. That's important for us to know, thank you.
7. OK, we'll have to remember that. Anything else you like doing?
8. I see you use a walking stick at home.
9. How about the rest of your mobility? Can you walk to the bathroom by yourself, for example, or do you need to use a commode?
10. You don't wear a hearing aid, so… not hard of hearing. But do you need glasses?

Communication Focus

It is the patient's right to decide the degree of involvement that their family or significant others have in their healthcare process.

In pairs, discuss the following questions.

1. Why do you think it is important to respect the patient's rights?
2. Assuming that the patient does want family members or significant others to involve in his/her care and decision-making, how should the nurse communicate with him/her?

Part One   Talking About Old Age

Task 1 **Work in pairs.**

Think of an elderly person you know well and how ageing has affected him/her. Think about the answers to these questions. Then talk to your partner about the person.

1. What daily tasks does he/she need to be helped with?

2. How does he/she keep mentally fit?

3. How does he/she keep physically fit?

4. What worries him/her?

5. How happy is he/she?

6. How healthy is he/she?

Task 2 **Complete and read.**

Label photos a-f with the aids in the box and try to match the useful sentences below.

| commode | dentures | glasses | grabber | hearing aid | walking frame |

a.＿＿＿＿＿＿＿

b.＿＿＿＿＿＿＿

c.＿＿＿＿＿＿＿

d.＿＿＿＿＿＿＿

e.＿＿＿＿＿＿＿

f.＿＿＿＿＿＿＿

Useful sentences:

1. Patients use a commode when they	a. hear better.
2. Patients wear dentures when they lose	b. up objects they cannot reach.
3. Patients wear glasses in order	c. are not able to walk to the toilet.
4. Patients use grabber to pick	d. them walk around more easily.
5. Patients wear hearing aid to	e. to see better.
6. Patients use walking frame to help	f. their natural teeth.

Task 3 **Listen and answer.** 🎧

Listen to a conversation between a nurse and Helen, a new care home resident, and answer the following questions.

1. What are Helen's hobbies?

2. Why doesn't Helen like TV?

3. How many children does Helen have?

4. Why is the Internet access so important for Helen?

Part Two Assessing an Elderly Care Home Resident

Task 4 **Listen and check.** 🎧

Listen to the first part of a conversation between a nurse and Devin Gyawali, a new care home resident, and choose the correct words in italics in this Assessment Form.

Assessment Form

Personal

- I would like to be called 1._____ *Mr. Gyawali/Devin.*
- I'm happy when 2._____ *I see my family/I'm by myself.*
- 3._____ *Impolite or unfriendly people/Noisy places* make me angry.
- My favourite foods are 4._____ *Spanish and French/Italian and Indian.*
- Foods I dislike are bananas and 5._____ *eggs/fish.*
- I 6._____ *wear/don't wear* dentures.

Task 5 Listen and complete. 🎧

Listen to the second part of the conversation and complete the rest of the Assessment Form.

Hobbies and interests

- My hobbies and interests are sports—1._____ and 2._____ and music—
  3._____ and 4._____ Indian music.
- I watch 5._____ on TV. I listen to 6._____ on the radio. I 7._____ magazines.

Mobility

- I use a(n) 8._____ and a(n) 9._____ to move around.
- I 10._____ to use a commode.
- I find it difficult to bend, so I use a(n) 11._____ to pick things up.

Communication

- I 12._____ hearing problems.
- I 13._____ eyesight problems, so I wear 14._____ .

Task 6 Role-play.

Student A is a new care home resident. Read Case Study 1 and complete this Assessment Form. Invent some of the information. Student B is a nurse who interviews Student A. Then swap roles and repeat the activity for Case Study 2.

Assessment Form

Personal

- I would like to be called 1._____.
- I'm happy when 2._____.
- 3._____ make(s) me angry.
- My favorite foods are 4._____.
- Foods I dislike are 5._____.
- I *wear/don't wear* dentures.

Hobbies and interests

- My hobbies and interests are 6._____.
- I *watch/don't watch* 7._____ (on) TV. I *listen/don't listen* to 8._____ (on)
  the radio. I *read/don't read* magazines.

Mobility

- I *use/don't use* a(n) 9._____ to move around.
- I *find it difficult/not difficult* to bend, so I *use/don't use* a 10._____ to pick things up.
- I *use/don't use* a commode.

Communication

- I *have/don't have* hearing problems, so I *wear/don't wear* 11._____ .
- I *have/don't have* eyesight problems, so I *wear/don't wear* 12._____ .

Case Study 1: Ms. Sandy Brown is 80 years old. She has hearing problems. She has difficulty in walking and needs to use a commode at night. She wears dentures.

Case Study 2: Mr. Dipak Clark is 92. He wears dentures and glasses. He also has poor hearing. He finds it difficult to walk without a walking frame. He needs to use a commode.

Part Three　Promoting Health of the Elderly

Task 7 **Work in pairs.**

Look at the illustrations a-j and write down facility (F) or activity (A) in the blanks. Then discuss with your partners which facilities and activities you think an ideal care home should have.

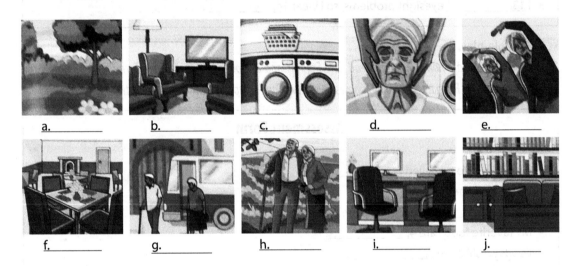

a._____　b._____　c._____　d._____　e._____

f._____　g._____　h._____　i._____　j._____

Task 8 **Listen and check.** 🎧

Listen to two elderly people in a care home talking and tick (√) the things that Julie (the first speaker) mentions.

Julie wants ...
☐ respect
☐ friends
☐ privacy
☐ to play bingo
☐ more stimulation
☐ to go to the seaside
☐ independence
☐ more food
☐ to go home

Julie doesn't like ...
☐ the staff
☐ Barbara
☐ her own name
☐ bingo
☐ coach trips
☐ her own home
☐ her old life
☐ the food
☐ washing up

Task 9 **Practice.**

Read the following passage and discuss with your partner about what you know about Alzheimer's disease. How does it affect a person in the following aspects?

1. Memory

2. Behaviour

3. Speech

4. Walking

5. Daily life

Alzheimer's disease damages the brain, destroying memory and reasoning. People with Alzheimer's disease suffer from confusion and loss of cognitive function. They need more and more nursing care as they become progressively more helpless, and finally die. The illness has three stages.

Early stage

1. forgetting recent conversations or events—Memory

2. minor changes in abilities and behaviour—Behaviour

3. repetition—Behaviour

Middle stage

1. needing some help with ADLs—Daily life

2. wandering—Walking

3. loss of interest in other people—Behaviour

4. unusual behaviour—Behaviour

5. shuffling gait—Walking

Later stage

1. needing constant help with ADLs—Daily life

2. forgetting names—Memory

3. complete loss of memory—Memory

4. inability to recognize familiar people, objects, or places—Memory

5. getting easily upset or aggressive—Behaviour

6. confusing night and day—Daily life

7. confinement to bed or a wheelchair—Walking

8. difficulty in swallowing—Daily life

9. loss of speech—Speech

More Practice

Role-play.

Read the following case and play the roles of a nurse and a patient based on the case. In the dialogue, you should complete the tasks below the case.

Case Study: Julie Green is a 65-year-old widow who has been suffering from COPD for 3 years and requires a long-term hospitalization. During her hospital stay, you find that no one has ever been visiting her. The patient is lonely and depressed. You are asked to encourage the patient to talk about her concerns.

Tasks:

1. Try to find out the reasons why she is lonely and depressed.
2. Find the persons who can visit the patient and make her happy.

New words

1. walking stick a stick carried in the hand for support in walking 手杖，拐杖
2. mobility / məʊˈbɪləti / *n.* the quality of moving freely 移动性
3. hearing aid a device which people with hearing difficulties wear in their ears to enable them to hear better 助听器
4. walking frame a tool for disabled or elderly people who need additional support to maintain balance or stability while walking 助行架
5. bingo /ˈbɪŋgəʊ / *n.* a game played for money or prizes, in which numbers are chosen by chance and called out, and if you have the right numbers on your card, you win 宾戈游戏
6. stimulation / ˌstɪmjuˈleɪʃn / *n.* the act of arousing an organism to action 刺激
7. Alzheimer's /ˈæltshaɪməz / disease a progressive form of presenile dementia that is similar to senile dementia except that it usually starts in the 40s or 50s; its first symptoms are impaired memory which is followed by impaired thought and speech and finally complete helplessness 阿尔茨海默氏痴呆；老年痴呆症
8. cognitive /ˈkɒgnətɪv / *adj.* relating to the mental process involved in knowing, learning, and understanding things 认识过程的；认知的
9. ADLs: the activities of daily living 日常生活活动
10. wander /ˈwɒndə(r) / *v.* to walk slowly across or around an area, usually without a clear direction or purpose 徘徊；闲逛
11. shuffle /ˈʃʌfl / *v.* to walk very slowly and noisily, without lifting your feet off the ground 拖着脚步走
12. gait / geɪt / *n.* the way someone walks 步态；步伐
13. aggressive / əˈgresɪv / *adj.* behaving in an angry and threatening way, as if you want to fight or attack someone 好斗的；挑衅的

14. confinement / kənˈfaɪnmənt / *n.* the act of putting someone in a room, prison etc. that they are not allowed to leave, or the state of being there 监禁；关押；禁闭

15. swallow /ˈswɒləʊ / *v.* to make food or drink go down your throat and towards your stomach 吞下；咽下（食物或饮料）

16. GP: general practitioner a doctor who is trained in general medicine and treats people in a particular area or town（在某一地区或城镇行医的）全科医生；普通医师

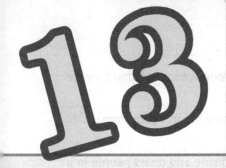

13 | Caring for Obstetric Patients

Intended Learning Objectives

On completion of the unit, students should be able to:

1. offer childbirth instructions;
2. provide delivery care for patients;
3. provide breastfeeding guidance.

Lead-in

Listen and repeat. 🎧

Listen to the following sentences and repeat them. Pay attention to the pronunciation and intonation.

1. Pregnancy is not a disease, and childbirth is the normal physiological result of completion of pregnancy.
2. Normal delivery can make the mother's womb recover more quickly and better.
3. Cesarean may make the newborn baby hard to breathe.
4. The baby can't be born until the cervix is fully dilated.
5. Open your mouth. Breathe quickly and shallowly.
6. When the next cramp comes, you can start pushing down, just like when you go to the toilet.
7. "Early sucking" means mother-infant skin contact and assists breastfeeding within half an hour after the baby's birth.
8. It is not only economic, simple and with proper temperature, but also helpful in increasing the baby's immune function, add the baby's anti-disease capability, and promote the growth of the baby's brain cells.
9. It can also help your uterus recovery, reduce post-partum bleeding, and reduce the chances of breast and ovarian cancer.
10. Let the baby's mouth cover your nipple and most of your areola.

Communication Focus

Active listening is an effective communication tool.

In pairs, discuss the following questions.

1. Why do you think active listening is an effective communication tool?
2. What do we need to do to develop the habit of active listening?

Part One   Waiting for Delivery

Task 1 **Work in pairs.**

Match the words to the meanings. Explain the words to your partner.

Example: *...stands for...; ...means...*

1. pregnant   a. the process of giving birth

2. placenta   b. a surgical operation for delivering a baby by cutting the walls of the mother's abdomen and womb

3. delivery   c. carrying developing offspring within the body

4. cramp   d. the temporary organ that feeds a fetus inside its mother's womb

5. backache   e. a painful and involuntary muscular contraction

6. cervix   f. the process of becoming wider or more open

7. cesarean   g. a pain in your back

8. dilatation   h. the narrow lower part of the womb that leads into the vagina

Task 2 **Pronounce the words.** 🎧

Write down the words according to the phonetic symbols below. And then listen and check.

1. / sɪˈzeərɪən / _____   2. /ˈpregnənsi / _____

3. /ˈjuːtərəs / _____   4. / wuːm / _____

5. / ˈæbdəmən / _____   6. /ˌdaɪleɪˈteɪʃn / _____

7. /ˈnɔːzɪeɪtɪd / _____   8. /ˌhaɪ ˈrɪsk / _____

Task 3 **Listen and write.** 🎧

Listen to the sentences and fill in the blanks with the right words.

1. Lying on the left side can increase the _____ between the uterus and the _____.

2. The fetus is in a _____ and the head is deep _____.

3. Do you feel the _____ regularly?

4. The _____ are coming more often and are lasting longer.

5. The _____ is open about three centimeters.

6. Your baby will be _____ soon.

Part Two   Delivery Care

Task 4 **Work in pairs.** 🎧

Put the following sentences in the correct order. Listen and check.

1. so, contractions, My, are, together, close.

2. dilated, fully, cervix, is, Your.

3. time, to, delivery, the, go, room, to, It's.

4. cramp, a, there, Is, coming?

5. breathe, and, shallowly, quickly, mouth, your, Open, and.

6. you, When, cramp, the, comes, next, pushing, start, down, can.

7. The, vagina, has, head, descended, the, into.

8. going, make, surgical, at, the, delivery, so, easier, be, will, perineum, small, a, incision, I'm, to, the.

Task 5 **Work in pairs.** 🎧

Discuss with your partner about how we divide the stages of labour. Then listen and fill in the blanks with the right words.

The first stage— 1._____: In this stage, and the woman is sociable and excited in latent phase, becoming more inwardly focused on the labour intension.

The second stage— 2._____: This is a pushing stage, and the woman has intense concentration on pushing, and may doze between contractions.

The third stage— 3._____: The woman is excited and relieved after her baby's birth. She is usually very tired.

The fourth stage— 4._____: 1 to 4 hours after the expulsion of the placenta, the woman is tired, but may find it difficult to rest because of the excitement and eager to be acquainted with the newborn.

Task 6 **Role-play.** 🎧

Play the role and listen to the sample.

Scenario: In the delivery room, the woman's cervix is fully dilated. It's time to go to delivery.

Task: Student A plays as a midwife, Student B plays as a nurse, both of them provide the delivery care for the woman. Student C plays as the woman who is a patient. And swap the roles later.

Useful sentence patterns:

1. Your cervix is fully dilated; it's time to go to the delivery room.

2. Open your mouth. Breathe quickly and shallowly.

3. When the next cramp comes, you can start pushing down.

4. Is there a cramp coming?

5. Wait until you can't hold it any longer and then start pushing down, just like when you go to the toilet.

6. Take a deep breath and push!

7. I see the baby's crown.

8. I'm going to make a small surgical incision at the perineum so delivery will be easier.

9. You shouldn't have any serious tears.

Part Three   Breastfeeding Guidance

Task 7 Listen and choose. 🎧

Listen to the dialogue and choose the correct suck posture. And then describe it to your partner.

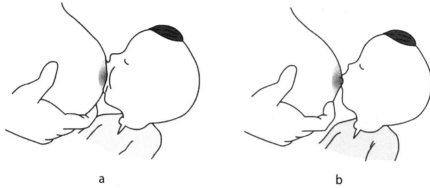

a   b

Task 8 Work in pairs.

Label the pictures of the feeding posture with the words below. And try to explain to your partner how to present the posture.

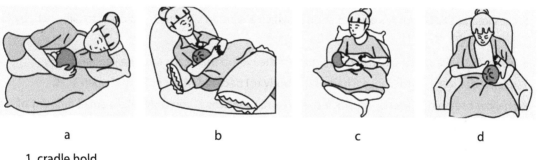

a   b   c   d

1. cradle hold _____

2. recline/laid-back _____

3. football hold_____

4. side-lying _____

Task 9 Questions and answers. 🎧

Listen to the dialogue, answer the following questions, and then report to the class.

1. What is "early sucking"?

2. What is the benefit of "early sucking"?

3. What can we do to stimulate the breast milk secretion?

4. What are the benefits of breastfeeding?

More Practice

Role-play.

Read the following case and play the roles of a nurse and a patient based on the case. In the dialogue, you should complete the tasks below the case.

Case Study: Li Mei is pregnant, and it's the firstborn. Her mother wants her to have caesarean birth, but her mother-in-law insists she should deliver normally.

Tasks:

1. Express your opinion about the problem.
2. Explain the benefits of normal delivery.

New words

1. delivery / dɪˈlɪvəri / *n.* a birth 分娩
2. breastfeed /ˈbrestfiːd / to feed a baby with milk directly from the mother's breasts 母乳喂养
3. pregnant /ˈpregnənt / *adj.* having a baby or babies developing inside the womb 怀孕的
4. womb / wuːm / *n.* 子宫（同 uterus）
5. caesarean / sɪˈzeəriən / *n.* an operation in which a woman's uterus is cut open to allow a baby to be born 剖腹产
6. cervix /ˈsɜːvɪks / *n.* the narrow lower part of the womb that leads into the vagina 子宫颈
7. dilate / daɪˈleɪt / *vi.* to (cause a part of the body to) become wider or further open 扩张
8. shallow breathing /ˈʃæləʊ ˈbriːðɪŋ / the breathing in which you only take a small amount of air into your lungs with each breath 浅呼吸
9. cramp / kræmp / *n.* a sudden painful tightening in a muscle 绞痛
10. suck / sʌk / *vt.* to pull in liquid or air through your mouth without using your teeth 吸吮
11. capability / ˌkeɪpəˈbɪləti / *n.* the ability to do something 能力
12. uterus /ˈjuːtərəs / *n.* the organ in the body of a woman or other female mammal in which a baby develops before birth 子宫
13. post-partum /ˌpəʊst ˈpɑːtəm / *adj.* occurring immediately after giving birth 产后的
14. ovary /ˈəʊvəri / *n.* either of the pair of organs in a woman's body that produce eggs 卵巢
15. nipple /ˈnɪpl / *n.* the dark part of the skin which sticks out from the breast of a mammal and through which milk is supplied to the young 乳头
16. areola / əˈriːələ / *n.* the circular area of darker skin around a nipple 乳晕
17. placenta / pləˈsentə / *n.* the temporary organ that feeds a fetus 胎盘
18. fetus /ˈfiːtəs / *n.* an animal or human being in its later stages of development before it is born 胎儿
19. vagina / vəˈdʒaɪnə / *n.* the part of a woman's body that connects her outer sex organs to her uterus 阴道
20. abdomen /ˈæbdəmən / *n.* the lower part of a person's body, containing the stomach, bowels,

and other organs, or the end of an insect's body 腹部

21. nauseated /'nɔ:zieɪtɪd / *adj.* feeling as if you are going to vomit 想吐的

22. contraction / kən'trækʃn / *n.* the fact of something becoming smaller or shorter 收缩

23. surgical incision /'sɜ:dʒɪkl ɪn'sɪʒn / an opening that is made in something with a sharp tool, especially in someone's body during an operation 手术切口

24. perineum /ˌperɪ'ni:əm / *n.* the area between the anus and the scrotum or vagina 会阴

25. efface / ɪ'feɪs / *vt.* to remove something intentionally 消除

26. expulsion / ɪk'spʌlʃn / *n.* squeezing out by applying pressure 排出

27. replace / rɪ'pleɪs / *vt.* to take the place of something, or to put something or someone in the place of something or someone else 替代

28. obstetric ward / əb'stetrɪk wɔ:d / relating to the area of medicine that deals with pregnancy and the birth of babies 产科病房

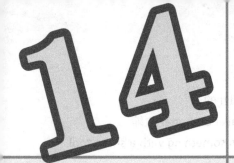

Helping Patients with Rehabilitation

Intended Learning Objectives

On completion of the unit, students should be able to:

1. understand some terms of rehabilitation;
2. help patients in ADLs;
3. instruct patients in recovery exercises;
4. praise patients in rehabilitation.

Lead-in

Listen and repeat.

Listen to the following sentences and repeat them. Pay attention to the pronunciation and intonation.

1. You did a good job. / Fabulous. / Good job. / Now you've got it. / You tried hard. / You are on top of it. / Super job.
2. You're improving. / You are on target. / You're on your way. / You're making progress.
3. Don't rush. / No rush. There's plenty of time.
4. Tell me if it hurts.
5. Your body needs the nutrition so that you can regain your strength and energy.
6. I have noticed that you have fought to recover in such a determined way.
7. It's common after the shock of such a big car accident.
8. Long stay in bed may make you lose confidence.
9. You have done very well considering the extent of your injuries.
10. I think we could stop here.

Communication Focus

Praise patients for their strengths and recovery progress.

In pairs, discuss the following questions.

1. Why do you think praising patients' strengths and recovery progress is important?
2. How will you praise your patients? List 3 sentences which could be used in such a conversation.

Part One   Introducing Rehabilitation Therapy

Task 1 **Work in pairs.**

Match the pictures with the terms below.

1. Occupational Therapy (   )

a method of helping people who have been ill or injured to develop skills or get skills back by giving them certain activities to do

2. Speech and Language Therapy (   )

the treatment of people who have speech and language problems

3. Physiotherapy (   )

a medical treatment for problems of the joints, muscles, or nerves, which involves doing exercise or having parts of the body massaged or warmed

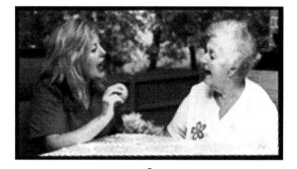

a

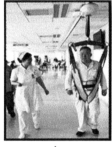

b

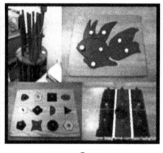

c

Task 2 **Pronounce the words.** 🎧

Write down the words according to the phonetic symbols below. And then listen and check.

1. / ˌɒkjʊˈpeɪʃənl / _____

2. /ˈθerəpi / _____

3. /ˈtriːtmənt / _____

4. /ˌfɪziəʊˈθerəpi / _____

5. / dʒɔɪnt / _____

6. /ˈmʌsl / _____

7. / nɜːv / _____

8. /ˈmæsɑːʒ / _____

Task 3 **Listen and check.** 🎧

Listen to the audio and complete the steps of guiding a patient in recovery exercises.

1) 1._____ the 2._____ and 3._____ of the exercise.

2) Set the 4._____ .

3) 5._____ the patient.

Part Two   Helping Patients in ADLs

Task 4 **Work in pairs.**

Label the pictures with the words below. And describe what each equipment is used to do.

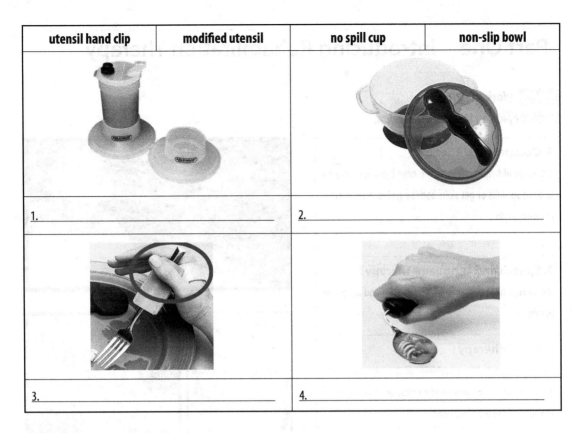

utensil hand clip	modified utensil	no spill cup	non-slip bowl
1.		2.	
3.		4.	

Task 5 Work in pairs. 🎧

Listen to a nurse helping Anita, a patient who is recovering from a stroke, with meal. Pay attention to the nurse's expressions of encouragement and comforting words used in the conversation, and put a tick (√) in the column. Then repeat it.

	1. It doesn't matter. / Never mind.
	2. Don't worry.
	3. I can really understand that you…
	4. You will recover soon.
	5. I could see that was hard work for you, but you did a good job.
	6. Don't be nervous. Your doctor is an expert for this disease.
	7. You did a good job. / You did really well.
	8. Please come back to see the doctor for a check-up in two weeks.

Task 6 Role-play.

Make a dialogue based on the following setting and play the role. You could take the audio scrip of Task 5 as a sample.

Scenario: in the ward

Instruments needed: a non-slip bowl, a no spill cup, some modified utensils

Task: Student A plays a ward nurse to help Student B, a patient recovering from a stroke, with meal. And swap the roles.

Useful sentence patterns:

1. Are you sitting up comfortably in the chair?

2. Don't rush. There's plenty of time.

3. Do you feel sick or uncomfortable?

4. I can really understand that you don't feel hungry.

5. Your body needs the nutrition so that you can regain your strength and energy.

6. Maybe you can try and eat on your own.

7. It's easier to hold.

8. I could see that was hard work for you. But you did a good job.

9. You should have a low-fat/low-salt/light/soft/liquid diet.

10. Please take more nutritious food.

Part Three   Instructing Patient in Rehabilitation

Task 7 Match pictures.

Match the pictures with the words below.

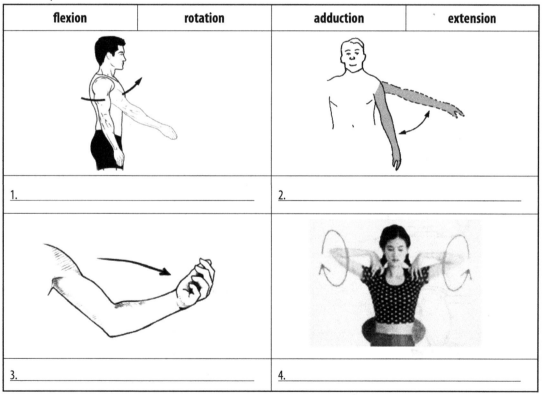

flexion	rotation	adduction	extension
1.		2.	
3.		4.	

Task 8 Listen and complete. 🎧

Listen and tick "√" the ROM exercises the patient can do in 1-6, and circle the correct words in 7-10.

<table>
<tr><td colspan="2">Flow sheet—ROM (range of motion exercise)</td><td>Patient: Theresa Smith
Room No.: Bed 64
Date: 21/11/2017
Time: 9:00 a.m.</td></tr>
</table>

Movement	Result	Comments
R shoulder flexion	1. _____	WNL (within normal limits)
R shoulder rotation	2. _____	WNL
R elbow extension	3. _____	7. WNL with some/no pain
R elbow flexion	4. _____	8. WNL with some/no pain
L shoulder flexion	5. _____	9. limited to 100°/120°
L shoulder extension	6. _____	10. able/not able to do
Nurse's initials	KPC	

Task 9 **Practice.**

Read the following case and practise encouraging a patient in recovery.

Task:

Student A is a nurse giving Student B, a patient, some instructions of the exercises for his knees and ankles.

Student B is an 18-year-old boy Hugo, who suffered from a car accident four months ago, and feels frustrated about the leg fracture.

Use the expressions in this table to help you.

	Ankle Pumps 1. Lay on bed and push your foot up and down slowly. 2. Eight or ten times a day.
	Ankle Rotations 1. Move your ankle in a circular motion. 2. Repeat 5 times in each direction. 3. Three or four times per day.
	Knee Bends 1. Keep heel on the bed and bend the knee. 2. Straighten the leg again. 3. Repeat 10 times. 4. Three or four times per day.

More Practice

Role-play.

Read the following case and play a nurse and a patient based on the flow sheet. In the dialogue, you should complete the tasks below the case.

Case Study: Mr. Carter is a 36-year-old man who works as a taxi driver. He suffered from a car accident three months ago and his right arm got fractured. He has a lovely 5-year-old son.

Flow sheet—ROM (range of motion exercises)		Patient: John Carter Room No.: Bed 19 Date: 18/7/2017 Time: 9: 00 a.m.
Movement	**Result**	**Comment**
R shoulder flexion	√	WNL (within normal limits)
R shoulder extension	√	limit 20°
R shoulder abduction	√	WNL
R shoulder adduction	√	WNL
Nurse's initials	GPR	

Tasks:

1. Guide the patient Mr. Carter through the range of motion exercises.

2. Praise the patient for his strength and recovery progress.

New words

1. rehabilitation /ˌriːəˌbɪlɪˈteɪʃn / *n.* the treatment of physical disabilities by massage, electrotherapy, or exercises 康复

2. recovery / rɪˈkʌvəri / *n.* the gradual healing after sickness or injury 痊愈；恢复

3. fabulous/ˈfæbjələs / *adj.* extremely good or impressive 令人难以置信的

4. rush / rʌʃ / *n.* the act of moving hurriedly and in a careless manner 匆忙 *v.* to move or to do sth. with great speed 迅速移动；匆忙地做

5. praise / preɪz / *v.* to say that you admire and approve of someone or something, especially publicly 赞美

6. occupational therapy / ˌɒkjuˈpeɪʃənl ˈθerəpi / a method of helping people who have been ill or injured to develop skills or get skills back by giving them certain activities to do 作业疗法

7. physiotherapy /ˌfɪziəʊˈθerəpi / *n.* a medical treatment for problems of the joints, muscles, or nerves, which involves doing exercises or having parts of your body massaged or warmed 物理疗法

8. joint / dʒɔɪnt / *n.* a part of your body such as your elbow or knee where two bones meet and are able to move together 关节

9. nerve / nɜːv / *n.* a network of long thin fibers that transmit messages between your brain and other parts of your body 神经

10. procedure / prəˈsiːdʒə(r) / *n.* a way of doing something, especially the correct or usual way 过程

11. slip / slɪp / *v.* to slide out of place or out of your hand 滑

12. bowl / bəʊl / *n.* a wide round container that is open at the top, used to hold liquids, food, flowers etc. 碗

13. tip / tɪp / *v.* to cause to topple or tumble by pushing 翻倒

14. modified /ˈmɒdɪfaɪd / *adj.* changed in form or character 改进的

15. utensil / juːˈtensl / *n.* a thing such as a knife, spoon etc. that you use when you are cooking 用具；厨具

16. flexion /ˈflekʃn / *n.* the act of bending a joint or limb 弯曲

17. rotation / rəʊˈteɪʃn / *n.* the act of turning with a circular movement around a central point 旋转

18. adduction / əˈdʌkʃn / *n.* moving of a body part toward the central axis of the body 内收

19. extension / ɪkˈstenʃn / *n.* the act of stretching or straightening out a flexed limb 扩展

20. elbow /ˈelbəʊ / *n.* the joint where your arm bends 肘

21. ankle /ˈæŋkl / *n.* the joint between your foot and your leg 脚踝

22. fracture /ˈfræktʃə(r) / *n.* a crack or break in something, especially a bone 骨折

23. abduction / æbˈdʌkʃn / *n.* the moving of a body part away from the central axis of the body 外展

Discharging Patients

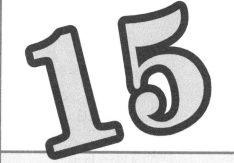

Intended Learning Objectives

On completion of the unit, students should be able to:

1. prepare patients for discharge;
2. give discharge instructions;
3. refer patients on the phone;
4. use appropriate English to communicate with patients, patients' relatives and other medical professionals.

Lead-in

Listen and repeat. 🎧

Listen to the following sentences and repeat them. Pay attention to the pronunciation and intonation.

1. Dr. Sim informed us that you were going home today, so I will remove your IV catheter and make a discharge plan for you.
2. It's a good idea to install grab bars around the bath, so she can hold on to them as she gets in and out of the bath.
3. If you get a raised toilet seat, you'll be able to slide from your wheelchair onto the toilet.
4. Lidia's daughter asked if you could let her know what time the home assessment's being done so she can come over to her mother's house.
5. The doctor has prescribed some medications for you; I just want to talk to you about them.
6. First, avoid any mental stress and have a good rest.
7. Secondly, examinations of fasting blood sugar and an ECG should be done regularly.
8. You need to keep the dressing on until you have your sutures removed.
9. I'm afraid I can't talk to you about your father's results because of confidentiality.
10. If you feel that there are any complications/problems, please contact the hospital immediately.

Communication Focus

"Turn-taking" in conversation is important and needs to be observed in a manner appropriate to the situation.

In pairs, discuss the following questions.

1. Why do you think "turn-taking" in conversation is important?
2. What do you usually do to improve your skill in "turn-taking" when talking with a patient?

Part One   Preparing Patients for Discharge

Task 1 **Work in pairs.**

To make a safe environment for the newly discharged patients, some mobility aids are needed at home. Label the pictures of mobility aids with the words below. Two students take turns to choose the item. One student explains what it is used for; the other student must guess the item.

Example (for pair work): *Student A: Something is used to help people to walk.*

Student B: It's a walking stick/walking frame.

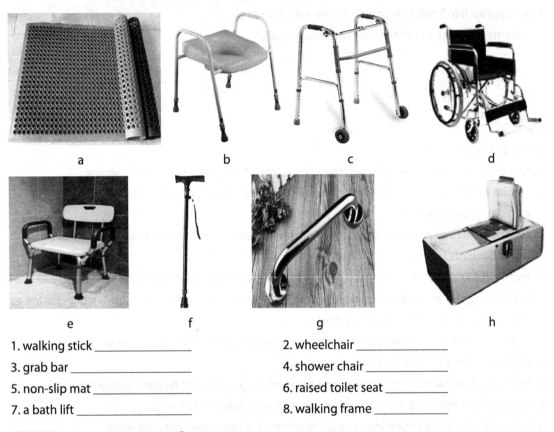

a   b   c   d

e   f   g   h

1. walking stick _____   2. wheelchair _____
3. grab bar _____   4. shower chair _____
5. non-slip mat _____   6. raised toilet seat _____
7. a bath lift _____   8. walking frame _____

Task 2 **Listen and complete.** 🎧

The discharged patient's current ADLs Assessment is a part of the Discharge Plan. Listen to a dialogue about a nurse going through a patient's Discharge Plan for the independence assessment. Tick (√) the correct boxes in the following assessment form.

ADLs Assessment				
Patient Name: Amy		**Ward:** 1		
Toileting	Independent ☐	Needs assistance ☐		Dependent ☐
Dressing	Independent ☐	Needs assistance ☐		Dependent ☐

ADLs Assessment			
Patient Name: Amy		**Ward:** 1	
Bathing/showering	Independent ☐	Needs assistance ☐	Dependent ☐
Eating	Independent ☐	Needs assistance ☐	Dependent ☐
Ambulation *	Independent ☐	Needs assistance ☐	Dependent ☐
Transferring **	Independent ☐	Needs assistance ☐	Dependent ☐

(**Note:** * getting around on foot   **getting around by vehicle)

Task 3 **Work in pairs.**

Preparing patients for discharge involves reading the discharge summary the doctor writes and reporting discharge summary to the colleagues at the ward team meeting. Study the following sample discharge summary. Find abbreviations in the chart for the following words. Then take turns to be the nurse giving brief report of the patient who will be discharged to the other student, using the following format.

Discharge Summary		
Patient: Linda Gilbert	**Sex:** female	**Age:** 80
HOD	2 weeks	
DOA	7th November 2018	
Attending Physician	Dr. John Hockings	
Conditions on Admission	left-sided weakness, difficulty in swallowing and speech	
AD	stroke (over the initial three hours from the onset of the stroke)	
Hospital Course	The patient was admitted and placed on aspirin, nutritive brain cell and intravenous fluid (to ensure the cerebral perfusion, nasal feeding and limb exercise).	
DOD	21th November 2018	
Conditions on Discharge	The patient improved, showing gradual resolution of left-sided weakness, swallowing and speech difficulties.	
DD	Stroke	
The patient is to follow up with Dr. John Hockings in one month. John Hockings D: 21/11/2018		

1. Date of Discharge   _____

2. Admitting Diagnosis   _____

3. Date of Admission   _____

4. Discharge Diagnosis   _____

5. Hospital Day   _____

Reporting format:

The patient is called…, and she is… years old. She was admitted because of…on (time)…. First, she was diagnosed as…and placed on…by attending physician Dr. John Hockings. After…days, the patient improved, showing gradual resolution of…. The patient will be discharged in a stable condition. Dr. Hockings prescribed some medications for her. Her follow-up appointment with Dr. Hockings has been made on…. (time and date) at Outpatient Department.

Part Two　Giving Discharge Instructions

Task 4 **Work in pairs.** 🎧

Put these words in order to make sentences. Discuss what the instructions are about by writing the number in the box below. Then listen and check.

1. already, sent, prescription, your, pharmacy, The, staff, nurse, has, to, the.

2. appointment, Let, with, me, check, follow-up, the, about, doctor, your.

3. regular, Have, keep, meals, vegetables, and, a, of, and, fruits, diet.

4. should, Which, take, I, exercise?

5. Your, Wednesday, been, follow-up, has, made, for, 10 a.m., appointment.

6. Continue, your, after, low-salt, your, diet, discharge.

7. mealtimes, Take, a, three, a, tablespoonful, day, at, times.

8. exercise, What, aerobic, are?

About exercise	About diet	About medication	About follow-up appointment

Task 5 **Work in pairs.** 🎧

The nurse is having conversations with three of her patients on their discharge. Listen to the three dialogues. What are the patients/caregivers worried about? Tick (√) the correct answer in the box below. What mobility aid(s) does the nurse recommend? Write down the answer in the right column. Then students work in pairs to have conversations about giving advice on mobility aids. Use the sentence patterns below to help you.

Dialogue	Patients/caregivers' worries			Nurse's advice about mobility aids
	bathing	toileting	dressing	
1				
2				
3				

You can begin like this (for pair work):

Nurse: So, do you think you are going to manage at home?/ Is there anything you are worried about?

Patient: Well, nurse, I am nervous about…/I have a problem…/ I just don't know how I can…

Nurse: Well, it's a good idea to…/ If you…, she will be able to …/ Why don't you…?

Patient: It sounds good. / Oh, it's a good idea. I'll try.

Task 6 **Role-play.**

Listen to the sample. Play the roles of the sample or play the roles following the role card below.

Scenario: in the ward

Instruments needed: a discharge form, some medicine, etc.

Task: Student A plays a nurse to give discharge instructions to Student B who plays a discharged patient. And swap the roles later.

Patient details			
Full Name:	*Margaret Williams*	**DOB:**	*15/10/1955*
DOA:	*10/3/2017*	**DOD:**	*14/3/2017*
Diagnosis:	*Hypertension*		
Discharge Instruction:	*1. Low-salt diet*		
	2. Rest, exercise		
	3. Oral medication: Lisinopril (赖诺普利，利压定) 10mg po daily		
	4. Continue to monitor BP		
	5. Follow-up appointment with Dr. Milton in a week		

Useful sentence patterns:

1. Here is a discharge form for you.

2. I can assure you'll fully recover after …

3. You should have a good rest for … and then go outdoors more, doing some exercise.

4. Keep a diet of …

5. Your doctor has written a prescription for you. Take …(dosage).

6. Continue to monitor your…

7. Remember to come to the Out-Patient Department for a consultation; your follow-up appointment with Dr. … is in …

8. You can pack your things and settle the account today.

9. We wish you an early recovery.

Part Three　Referring Patients on the Phone

Task 7 Work in pairs.

Ward staff often need to make telephone referrals to allied health departments or services. Complete the table below using the sentences in the box. Then ask each other questions and give answers.

Example： *Student A: How will you say who you are?*

Student B: ….

Sally speaking.
Could you please spell that for me?
I'd like to make a referral.
Do you want me to give you her daughter's number?
It's Tina calling.
I'd like to refer an 80-year-old lady to you for some District Nursing Services.
Does she need her meals delivered to her at home?
Could you hold for a minute?

Saying who you are	
Saying why you are calling	
Asking someone to do something	
Inquiring about something	

Task 8 Listen and complete. 🎧

Sandy, the Ward Nurse, makes a telephone referral to the District Nursing Service on a patient's discharge. Listen to the conversation and complete the sections marked 1-10.

Telephone Referral Form	
Service referred to	District Nursing Service
Name of patient	Linda 1.＿＿＿＿＿＿＿
Address	15 Summer Lane, Exeter
Entry to home (circle)	Digital Code/Key
	If by key, name of the caregiver with spare key: 2.＿＿＿＿

Phone number	3. _____
GP	Dr. John 4. _____
Referred by	Sandy Clarke (RN)
Place of referral	Alexandra Hospital
Diagnosis	stroke, mod. Left-sided weakness, difficulty in swallowing
Assistance with ADLs (circle)	5. bathing/mobility/nutrition
Diet (circle)	6. normal/soft/diabetic Other requirements (cultural/religious)
Delivery of meals (circle)	7. Yes/No
Home assessment booked (circle)	8. Yes/No If Yes, date booked: 9. _____
Aids/Equipment (circle if need to be ordered)	10. walking frame/shower chair/oxygen nebuliser
Next of kin	Andrea (daughter)
Phone number	0-145-667-9998

Task 9 Role-play. 🎧

Listen to the telephone conversation again and play the roles, using the information in the chart above.

Student A plays the Ward Nurse to make a referral for District Nursing Service.

Student B plays the District Nurse. And swap the role later.

Useful sentence patterns:

1. It's Sandy here from Alexandra Hospital.

2. I've got an 80-year-old lady. I'd like to refer to you for some District Nursing Services. Can I give you the details now?

3. Her address is 15 Summer Lane, Exeter.

4. The spare key is with her daughter, Andrea. Her daughter is also her next of kin.

5. She had a stroke two weeks ago. And she needs quite a lot of help with her ADLs, especially bathing and mobility.

6. I think it's better to have a home assessment done.

7. Does she need any aids? Do I have to order a walking frame for her?

8. How has she managed with her diet?

9. Does she need her meals delivered to her at home?

10. Is there anything else you need to know?

More Practice

Role-play.

Read the following case and play a nurse and the patient's next of kin based on the case. In the dialogue, you should complete the tasks below the case.

Case Study: Eric Blake, a 75-year-old retired railway worker, who has been living in his own home for 25 years, suffered a stroke two weeks ago. When he was sent to hospital he had right-sided weakness, swallowing and speech difficulties. It was well over the initial three hours from the onset of the stroke. He has been in hospital for two weeks. Now he shows gradual resolution and is ready to be discharged. You are the Charge Nurse, Kathy, after having a weekly team meeting which is on Eric, the discharged patient's care, talks to Wendy, his daughter on his discharge.

Tasks:

1. Explain the effects of a stroke.
2. Inform the patient of what you've been doing.
3. Give advice on the care at home.

New words

1. discharge / dɪsˈtʃɑːdʒ / v. to officially allow someone to leave somewhere, especially the hospital 出院
2. catheter /ˈkæθɪtə(r) / n. a thin tube that is put into your body to remove liquids 导液管
3. install / ɪnˈstɔːl / v. to put a piece of equipment somewhere and connect it so that it is ready to be used 安装
4. dressing /ˈdresɪŋ / n. a special piece of material used to cover and protect a wound 敷料
5. suture /ˈsuːtʃə(r)/ n. a stitch that is used to sew a wound together 缝针
6. complication / kɒmplɪˈkeɪʃn / n. a medical problem or illness that happens while someone is already ill and makes treatment more difficult 并发症
7. mat / mæt / n. a piece of thick soft material used in some activities for people to sit on 垫子
8. frame / freɪm / n. the structure or main supporting parts of a piece of furniture, vehicle, or other objects 架子
9. ambulation / æmbjʊˈleɪʃn / n. walking about 移动；步行
10. transfer / trænsˈfɜː(r)/ v. to move around 转移
11. anticoagulate / æntikəʊˈægjʊleɪt / v. to prevent from becoming thick and almost solid（尤指用抗凝血剂）防止……凝血
12. cerebral / səˈriːbrəl / adj. of the brain 大脑的
13. perfusion / pəˈfjuːʒən / n. pumping a liquid into an organ or tissue (especially by way of blood vessels）灌注；充满
14. resolution /ˌrezəˈluːʃn / n. solution 解决
15. aerobic / eəˈrəʊbɪk / adj. requiring air or free oxygen for life 需氧的
16. frail / freɪl / adj. physically weak 虚弱的
17. buzzer /ˈbʌzə(r)/ n. a small thing, usually shaped like a button, that buzzes when you press it 蜂鸣器；按铃
18. nourishment /ˈnʌrɪʃmənt / n. the food and other substances that people and other living things need to live, grow, and stay healthy 营养品

19. consultation /ˌkɒnslˈteɪʃn / *n.* a meeting with a professional person, especially a doctor, for advice or treatment 会诊

20. referral / rɪˈfɜːrəl / *n.* referring or being referred to sb./sth. 送交

21. ally /ˈælaɪ / *v.* to join or become joined with sb./sth. by treaty, marriage, etc. 结盟

22. bungalow /ˈbʌŋɡələʊ / *n.* a small house that is built all on one level 平房

23. moderate (mod.) /ˈmɒdərət / *adj.* not excessive or extreme 温和的

24. diabetic / ˌdaɪəˈbetɪk / *adj.* of or relating to or causing diabetes 糖尿病的

25. nebuliser /ˈnebjulaɪzə / *n.* a dispenser that turns a liquid (such as perfume) into a fine mist 喷雾器

26. adaption /ˌəˈdæpʃn / *n.* the act of changing something or changing your behaviour to make it suitable for a new purpose or situation 适应

References

陈仁英，高芸，2008. 护理英语口语. 上海：上海科学技术出版社.

陈迎，2014. 新职业英语行业篇——医护英语. 北京：外语教学与研究出版社.

弗吉尼娅，帕特里西娅，2010. 护理英语1. 北京：中国青年出版社.

弗吉尼娅，帕特里西娅，2010. 护理英语2. 北京：中国青年出版社.

雷子强，2007. 西方临床护理英语全攻略. 北京：北京大学医学出版社.

刘国全，2006. 护理专业英语——视听说分册. 北京：人民卫生出版社.

刘国全，2008. 护理英语学习指导. 北京：人民卫生出版社.

帕金林，克里斯，2006. 国际护士日常英语. 北京：人民卫生出版社.

沈海燕，2012. 新编国际护理英语——听说教程. 北京：北京大学医学出版社.

沈洁，2005. 高级护理英语教程——口语分册. 上海：上海科学技术出版社.

史冬梅，2016. 护理职业交际英语. 上海：复旦大学出版社.

王文秀，王颖，2011. 英汉对照护理英语会话. 北京：人民卫生出版社.

谢红，李晓玲，2005. 护理专业英语. 四川：四川大学出版社.

徐淑秀，李建群，2005. 实用护理英语. 北京：人民军医出版社.

徐小贞，2015. 新职业英语（第二版）行业篇医护英语. 北京：外语教学与研究出版社.

张凤军，白兴武，2000. 临床护理英语. 北京：中国对外经济贸易出版社.

朱红梅，毕向群，2015. 护理英语. 北京：人民卫生出版社.

朱琦，2005. 国际护理考试（NCLEX）护理英语9（中级）. 上海：上海科学技术文献出版社.

ALEXANDER G C, MOHAJIR N, MELTZER D O, 2005. Consumers' Perceptions about Risk of and Access to Nonprescription Medications. Journal of the American Pharmacists Association, 45(3).

ALLUM V, MCGARR P, 2008. Cambridge English for Nursing Intermediate. UK: Cambridge University Press.

FIELD L, SMITH B, 2008. Nursing Care. UK: Pearson Education Limited.

GRICE T, 2011. Nursing 1. UK: Oxford English for Careers.

GRICE T, GREENAN J, 2013. Nursing 2. UK: Oxford English for Careers.

WRIGHT R, CAGNOL B, SYMONDS M S, 2017. English for Nursing 1. UK: Pearson Education Limited.

WRIGHT R, CAGNOL B, SYMONDS M S, 2017. English for Nursing 2. UK: Pearson Education Limited.

Audio Script

Unit 1

Lead-in

Listen and repeat.

Listen to the following sentences and repeat them. Pay attention to the pronunciation and intonation.

1. Good morning, Mr. Brown. My name is Cindy. I'll be the nurse looking after you today.

2. Would you mind if I ask you a few questions? / We need some information from you.

3. Can you tell me your full name and the date of birth, please?

4. I'd like to know why you're here today.

5. Do you have any allergies to medications?

6. Can you tell me the name of your next of kin?

7. I'd like to know the phone number of your next of kin.

8. What is your job? / Could you tell me your occupation?

9. Do you have any serious illnesses in the past?

10. Please wait a moment. I'll let your doctor know. / I'll inform your doctor.

Task 2 Pronounce the words.

Write down the words according to the phonetic symbols below. And then listen and check.

1. emergency	2. pediatrics	3. surgery
4. maternity	5. geriatrics	6. radiology

Task 3 Listen and complete.

Listen to the following sentences carefully and fill in the missing words. Then read the sentences with your partner.

1. Pediatric Dept. is where they treat children.

2. Surgical Dept. is where surgeons carry out operations.

3. Emergency Room is the place where they treat emergency cases.

4. Radiology Dept. is where they take X-rays.

5. Midwives deliver babies in the Maternity Unit.

6. Specialists in geriatrics treat problems related to the elderly.

Task 4 Work in pairs.

Put the following sentences in the correct order and then listen to the conversation and check your answer.
Sample:

(S=Sarah, nurse; G=Mr. Green, patient)

S: Good morning, Mr. Green. My name is Sarah, I'm in charge of this ward. If you need anything, please press this button.

G: Good morning, Sarah. Could you tell me the hours here for having meals and visiting?

S: Sure. Patients usually get up at 7: 00 a.m. Breakfast is at 8: 00 a.m. The ward rounds and treatment start at 9 a.m. After lunch you could have a nap or rest. Visiting hours are from 3: 00 p.m. to 7: 00 p.m. Supper is at 6 p.m. Bed time is from 9: 30 p.m. to 10: 00 p.m. And we provide hot water 24 hours.

G: Thank you. Will you show me where the bathroom is?

S: Of course, it is over there at the corner. And do you need clean pajamas?

G: Yes, please. Is it possible for my family to stay here with me?

S: We don't think it is necessary, since your condition isn't so serious.

G: OK. That's fine.

S: Please let us know if you need any help, and smoking is not allowed here.

Task 5 Work in pairs.

Put these words in order to make sentences. Discuss the details of one patient which the nurse should take down in admission. Listen and check your answers.

1. Good morning, Caroline. I'm sorry to trouble you so much.

2. Welcome, Mrs. Johnson. I'm Daisy, the nurse in charge of this department.

3. Would you mind if I check out some details of you?

4. What would you like to know?

5. I'd like to check your name and date of birth.

6. My full name is Catherine Jonathan and the date of my birth is the fifth of July nineteen fifty seven.

7. I'll bring you to your bedside. Please follow me.

8. We supply hot water and the toilet is over there.

9. Please let us know if you need any help.

10. Smoking is not allowed here.

Task 6 Role-play.

Play the role and listen to the sample.

Sample:

(N=nurse; P=patient)

N: Good morning Madam, I'd like to check your personal details, is that okay?

P: Yes, of course.

N: Could you tell me your full name, please?

P: Catherine Miller.

N: Can you spell that, please?

P: C-A-T-H-E-R-I-N-E, Catherine, M-I-L-L-E-R, Miller.

N: All right, and what would you like us to call you?

P: Catherine is fine.

N: Well, Catherine, where are you from?

P: I'm originally from Chicago. But I came here for my studies. I got married, and now I'm looking forward to my first child. I've been here for ten years already.

N: That's lovely, and what is your date of birth?

P: The 20th of August,1982.

N: Is that the 20th of August,1982?

P: That's right.

N: And what is your job?

P: Advertising manager for Bxx company.

N: Advertising manager. Okay, I also need to ask who your next of kin is, to contact in an emergency.

P: My husband, Daniel Miller, is my next of kin. His mobile number is 0677-998-7787.

N: Thank you. Do you have any allergies?

P: No.

Task 8 Listen and complete.

Listen to the audio and complete the chart. And act it out in pairs.

Sample:

(S=Sandy, nurse; C=Mr. Cooper, patient)

S: Mr. Cooper, have you got an ID bracelet on?

C: Yes, here it is.

S: I just need to check your personal details. Can I look at your ID bracelet, please?

C: Certainly.

S: Can you tell me your full name, please?

C: Allen Cooper.

S: Allen, A-L-L-E-N; Cooper, C-O-O-P-E-R. Right, that's correct on the bracelet. What's your date of birth, please?

C: The 20th of August, 1947.

S: The 20th of August, 1947. Now your hospital number is, seven, six, seven, eight, three, seven. I'll just check that on the identity bracelet. Well, that's correct.

C: Then, anything else?

S: One more question. Do you have any allergies?

C: Yes I do. I'm allergic to penicillin. It makes me very sick.

S: Oh, if you are allergic to something, you should have a red identity bracelet. I'll change that for you right away.

C: Oh, thanks, Sandy. I forgot to tell them about the allergy.

S: That's okay, Mr. Cooper. That's why we like to check everything carefully. And can you tell me the name of your next of kin?

C: It's my daughter, Katherine Cooper.

S: Can you tell me her telephone number?

C: Sure. Nine, four, seven, seven, zero, zero, seven, seven, five , seven, nine.

S: Okay, that's all for me.

C: Thanks, Sandy.

Unit 2

Lead-in

Listen and repeat.

Listen to the following sentences and repeat them. Pay attention to the pronunciation and intonation.

1. I'm just going to do your observations, is that OK?

2. Mr. Blake in bed 301 is now in rapid AF (atrial fibrillation). Can you please put him onto hourly obs.?

3. Please put this thermometer under your armpit for a short while, and keep your arm firmly up against your chest until I take it out.

4. The normal range for the body temperature is around 36 to 37 °C .

5. I'm just going to take your pulse. Can I have your wrist, please?

6. Hello Betty, Paul Miller in bed 15 is quite tachycardic. His heart rate is 130 but he is still in a regular sinus rhythm.

7. Before I take your blood pressure, could you please tell me if you have had any previous surgery done on either your chest or arms?

8. When I inflate the blood pressure cuff, it'll be a little tight.

9. His Resps. (respirations) were 18 at 14: 00.

10. Mrs. Chan still remains quite tachypnoeic most of the time, at a rate of 35.

Task 2 Pronounce the words.

Write down the words according to the phonetic symbols below. And then listen and check.

1. heart rate   2. pulse   3. blood pressure   4. respiratory

5. temperature   6. oxygen   7. saturation   8. observation

Task 3 Read aloud and check.

Read the following measurements and put a tick (√) in the correct column. And then listen to the audio and check.

1. one hundred and thirty-five millimetres of mercury

2. thirty-six point seven degrees Celsius

3. seventy-five beats per minute

4. twenty breaths per minute

5. ninety-eight point six degrees Farenheit

Task 5 Work in pairs.

Put these words in order to make sentences. Discuss which vital sign the nurse is taking in each case. Listen and check your answers.

1. Can you hold your arm out straight for me?

2. Just pop this under your tongue.

3. I'll put this probe into your ear.

4. Can I have your wrist, please?

5. Can you roll up your sleeve?

6. Please put your finger into this probe.

7. Just breathe in and out normally.

8. Can you give me your right hand, please?

Task 6 Role-play.

Play the role and listen to the sample.

Sample:

N: Ms. Smith, I'm going to take your obs. now. Is that OK?

P: Sure, go ahead.

N: Did you drink any hot water in the last half an hour?

P: No, I didn't.

N: OK, let me take your temperature first. Please put this thermometer under your armpit for a short while; and keep your arm firmly up against your chest until I take it out.

P: (*Takes the thermometer and puts it under the armpit.*) Is that right?

N: Yes, good. Have you been smoking, drinking coffee or taking any kind of stimulants today?

P: No, I haven't.

N: Well, I'm just going to take your pulse; can I have your wrist, please?

P: (*Stretches the arm on the table.*)

N: (*Looks at the watch and counts the pulse and respiration. And after finishing measuring them, writes down the readings.*)

P: How is my pulse?

N: Your pulse is sixty-five beats per minute. And I've also checked your respiration. It is eighteen breaths per minute.

P: Are they normal?

N: Yes, they are quite normal. Now, please give me the thermometer.

P: Here you are. Do I have a temperature?

N: (*Writes down the number on the chart.*) It is thirty-eight point three degrees Celsius, a little high. Before I take your blood pressure, could you please tell me if you have had any previous surgery done on either your chest or arms?

P: No.

N: Do you have any history of high blood pressure?

P: No, never.

N: Ok. Ms. Smith, please roll up the sleeve of your left arm, and lift your arm a little so I can put on the blood pressure cuff.

P: (*Rolls up the sleeve and lifts the arm on the table.*)

N: (*Wraps the cuff around the arm and then inflates the cuff.*) When I inflate the blood pressure cuff it'll be a little tight. (*Notes down the measurement on the chart.*) Your blood pressure is good, one hundred over eighty; it's in the normal range.

P: That's good.

N: All right. That's all for me. I'll report all the results to the doctor.

P: Thank you, nurse.

N: You are welcome.

Task 7 Work in pairs.

Look at the graphs and try to describe the changes of vital signs. And then listen to the audio and match each graph to the patient.

Patient 1: His resps. varied between ten and twenty-five.

Patient 2: Her temp. was up and down all night, but now it's stable at thirty-seven point five.

Patient 3: He was running a fever, but his temp.'s back to normal now.

Patient 4: Her pulse rate was extremely low, but now it's up to seventy.

Patient 5: His blood pressure went up from one hundred and twenty over eighty to one hundred and sixty over one hundred.

Patient 6: Her heart rate fell to twenty, but now it's rising again.

Task 8 Listen and complete.

Listen to the audio and complete the chart. And act it out in pairs.

(S=Susan, charge nurse; J=Jenifer, ward nurse.)

S: Jenifer, can you bring us up to date on Felton?

J: Felton Carter? Sure. As you know he was admitted just before 2: 00 a.m. today with poorly managed hypertension. He was put on four hourly obs. as Doctor Wang ordered. If you look at his Obs. Chart from today, you'll see that he was quite hypertensive on admission. BP was one hundred and seventy-five over one hundred and two, pulse eighty-six. At 6: 00 a.m., his BP was about the same, one seventy-six over ninety-five and pulse seventy-six. During the morning shift at 10: 00 a.m. he shot up to two hundred and ten over one thirty, with a pulse of a hundred and twelve. He had some chest pain, too. Doctor Wang came up to see him about the chest pain and high BP. He did all the usual things for his ECG, GTN sublingually, and he settled a bit by 2: 00 p.m. By 2: 00, his BP was one eighty-five over ninety and his pulse was ninety-seven. I took his obs. again at 3: 00 p.m., just before handover. He's gone down to one seventy over eighty-five with a pulse of eighty-six.

S: How was his Temp. and Resps.?

J: His Temp. was thirty-six five on admission and remained stable. His Resps. were up and down. They varied between sixteen and twenty-two, with the peak at 10: 00 a.m.

S: Thanks, Jenifer. We'll keep an eye on him.

J: All right, now I'll just let you know about Mrs. Castle.

S: Go ahead.

J: Rosa Castle's on hourly resps. She had a history of respiratory problems, and she became quite breathless after her operation today.

S: How's her respiratory rate now?

J: Um, you can see her pre-op Resps. at 6: 00 a.m. were eighteen. That's about normal for her. I checked her Resps. at 7: 00 a.m. before she went to operating theatre and they were still eighteen.

S: Mm. When did she come back from the operation?

J: She came back a couple of hours ago at, um, 2: 00 p.m. She was in a lot of pain and she was quite breathless. Her Resps. went up to twenty-six. I started her on some oxygen at five liters per minute for an hour between 2: 00-3: 00 p.m.

S: OK. I see. It looks like she's settled down a bit since then.

J: Yeah, I just did her obs. a few minutes ago at 3: 00 p.m. and her Resps. were down to twenty so that's better.

S: OK. We'll keep an eye on her, too.

Unit 3

Lead-in

Listen and repeat.

Listen to the following sentences and repeat them. Pay attention to the pronunciation and intonation.

1. What seems to be the trouble?

2. Please show me where the pain is.

3. Do you feel short of breath and are there any changes in your vision?

4. Does the pain spread anywhere else?

5. Have you had any nausea and vomiting?

6. How about your bowel movement and exhaust?

7. Have you noticed any blood in your motions/in your sputum/when you pass water?

8. Do you get a pain in your chest when you cough?

9. Have you noticed any coffee grounds, bile and blood in your vomit?

10. Did you run a fever or have a sore throat?

Task 1 Work in pairs.

Look at the following pictures and try to describe the symptoms. And then listen to the 10 patients describing their symptoms and match them to the pictures a-j.

1. I have had a severe stomachache for a few days.

2. I have a runny nose.

3. It hurts just behind my kneecap.

4. I have a sore throat and swollen glands.

5. I have an aching feeling in my shoulder, and tingling in my fingers.

6. I don't have any appetite.

7. I have red, blotchy rashes all over my body. They itch a lot.

8. I feel sweaty.

9. I have been feeling a little breathless.

10. I have a fever.

Task 2 **Work in pairs.**

Match 1-5 to a-e to make questions. Then listen and check your answer.

N: How long have you had the pain in your belly?

P: Since last night, it started around the umbilicus, but moved to the right this morning.

N: Has it moved again?

P: No. It has been steady for 4 hours.

N: Does the characteristic of the pain change?

P: It started as a blunt pain, but changed to a sharp pain, so severe that I can hardly stand it.

N: Have you had any diarrhea?

P: No. I haven't had any bowel movement for 2 days.

N: Did you have a fever?

P: Last night I took my temperature. It was 38 degrees Celsius.

Task 5 **Listen and complete.**

Listen to the nurse interviewing Mrs. Smith and check your answers in Task 4. Listen again and complete the patient record.

N: What brings you here?

P: I suffer from a bad headache.

N: Is it worse in the morning or evening?

P: It is severe in the morning.

N: In which part of the head do you feel the pain?

P: The pain is concentrated on the left part.

N: Do you ever feel sick?

P: Yes, it is accompanied by the headache in the morning.

N: Does the light hurt your eyes?

P: No.

N: Have you noticed any blurring of vision?

P: Yes, sometimes.

N: Do you ever see things double?

P: No.

N: Do you ever see flashing lights?

P: Yes, I see flashing lights three times.

N: Any other trouble with your eyes?

P: No.

N: Have you had any fits, faints or funny turns?

P: Yes, I have had fits these days.

N: Was there any warning that you were going to have a fit?

P: Last time I felt dizzy before the fit.

N: Did you bite your tongue?

P: Never.

N: Did you wet yourself?

P: No.

N: Do you have any problems with your hearing?

P: The hearing is worse than ever.

N: Have you noticed any numbness, tingling or weakness in your limbs?

P: I have numbness in my limbs. But it is irregular.

N: Do you pass more water than you used to?

P: No, I haven't noticed that.

Task 6 Role-play.

Play the role and listen to the sample.

(N=nurse; M=mother; C=child)

Sample:

M: My child has a temperature, a headache, a sore throat and a rash.

N: How long has he been ill?

M: He's had the temperature since yesterday.

N: Are there any sick children in the neighborhood or at school?

M: One of his classmates had a fever and complained of a sore throat five days ago.

N: (*Turns to the child*) Let me have a look. Open your mouth and show me your tongue. Say Ah…

C: Ah.

N: (*Uses the tongue depressor and the penlight to check the child's mouth.*) Now take off your clothes.

M: What have you found?

N: His tonsils are swollen and red. His tongue is as red as a strawberry. There is a rash all over his body.

N: He may need a blood test. Go to the Pathology Department for it and bring the result here, please.

(*Thirty minutes later.*)

M: Here is the result. Is it normal?

N: His white blood cell count is high. He is probably suffering from scarlet fever.

M: What kind of disease is it?

N: It is a kind of infectious disease. You should keep him away from other children as much as possible.

M: What can I do for him?

N: He should stay in bed until his fever goes down. Let him eat easily digestible food and drink plenty of fluid.

M: Does he need to take some drugs?

N: I'll tell the doctor and he will prescribe penicillin injections for a few days.

M: What should I do about his rash?

N: You should prevent him from scratching it.

M: OK. Thank you.

Unit 4

Lead-in

Listen and repeat.

Listen to the following sentences and repeat them. Pay attention to the pronunciation and intonation.

1. I will collect your blood to make sure what caused the fever.

2. Please roll up your sleeve, and lay your arm on the table.

3. I will sterilize your skin and tie the tourniquet around your arm.

4. I need to change the specimen tube. Please clench your fist.

5. I'm going to collect your urine to do a urinalysis.

6. I have brought you a urinal—this bottle. Please pass urine into it.

7. Please get some of your stools with this little spoon and put it back into the tube.

8. Please avoid getting any other things into the tube.

9. Otherwise it might give us a false result.

10. I will send the specimen to the lab. / I will do the test in the ward. The specimen won't be sent to the lab.

Task 2 Work in pairs.

Listen and match each sample collected with facts as its targets. Then explain the purposes of collecting each sample to your partner.

1. Urine test can provide information for a doctor about the infection in the kidneys or bladder.

2. Blood test can be ordered to look for signs of diabetes or liver inflammation.

3. Stool is tested when a doctor suspects a problem in the intestine.

Task 3 Pronounce the words.

Write down the words according to the phonetic symbols below. And listen to check.

1. urine	2. diabetes	3. stool	4. feces
5. intestine	6. infection	7. bladder	8. kidney

Task 5 Work in pairs.

Complete this dialogue about taking a blood sample from a 9-year-old boy with words in Task 4. Then listen and act it out in pairs.

Nurse: Good morning gentlemen. I'm Kelly. I will collect your blood to make sure what caused the fever. You are Calvin Green, right?

Patient: Yes…I don't like blood test! That's painful!

Nurse: If you follow my instructions, I promise, I will do it as gently as I can. Shall we? (*A big smile*)

Patient: …Ok, I will try.

Nurse: Please roll up your sleeve, and lay your arm on the table. I will sterilize your skin. Now I'm going to tie this tourniquet around your arm. Do you feel a small pin prick?

Patient: Yes, it's tight.

Nurse: It won't take long. May I know the name of your school?

(Distracts his attention and inserts the needle.)

Patient: I'm from No. 1 primary school…

Nurse: I see…now I need to change the specimen tube. Please clench your fist.

Patient: Oh…I feel dizzy…

Nurse: That will be fine. Be relaxed. Press here with cotton stick for a minute. I will send the specimen to the lab.

Patient: I don't feel well.

Nurse: You may take a rest on the couch. Maybe it will help you.

Patient: Thank you.

Nurse: How do you feel now?

Patient: I feel better. Thank you.

Task 6 **Role-play.**

Put these words in 1-16 in the correct order to make sentences and listen to the sentences and check the answer. Then use these sentences to make dialogues about collecting urine or stool and act it out.

Setting 1:

1. I'm going to collect your urine to do a urinalysis.

2. It can indicate problems in kidneys.

3. I have brought you a urinal—this bottle.

4. Please pass urine into it.

5. I will use a disposable dipstick to make sure there is protein or blood in the urine specimen.

6. It only takes several minutes.

7. I will do the test in the ward.

8. The specimen won't be sent to the lab.

9. Please ring when it is ready.

Setting 2:

10. Next time you open your bowels we need to collect your stool to do a stool test.

11. It can indicate problems in the intestine.

12. Here is a stool collection tube with spoon on the lid.

13. Please get some of your stools with this little spoon and put it back into the tube.

14. Please avoid getting any other things into the tube.

15. Otherwise it might give us a false result.

16. Please ring when it is ready.

Task 8 Listen and complete.

Listen to the audio and match the report with the patient.

Patient 1: Her urine is dark red and the pH is normal. Her urine is positive for white blood cell, protein and occult blood.

Patient 2: Her white blood cell is 12.5 billion per liter, and her hemoglobin is 130 grams per liter.

Patient 3: His stool has been soft or watery. His stool is positive for white blood cell, red blood cell and occult blood.

Task 9 Practice in pairs.

Listen and mark down the professional and laypersons' English for each Chinese term. Then act it out in pairs. Then practice the task below with your partner.

A. Blood Test

Nurse: (turns to patient)

Nurse: Morning, Mrs. Brown. How long have you had a cough?

Patient: More than one week.

Nurse: Are you coughing up any sputum?

Patient: Yes, I'm coughing up large amount of very sticky green phlegm.

Nurse: (turns to doctor)

Nurse: Doctor, Mrs. Brown reports she coughs up a lot of tenacious purulent sputum.

Doctor: How is her blood test?

Nurse: Her white blood cell is 12.5 billion per liter, and her hemoglobin is 130 grams per liter.

Doctor: It looks like she has RTI (respiratory tract infection). She'd better have an X-ray.

Nurse: Ok, I will inform her.

B. Urine Report

Nurse: (turns to patient)

Nurse: Mrs. Anita Ford, have you recently noticed anything unusual about your urine?

Patient: Yes. I pee more often than usual and it's painful. What's worse, as soon as I get the urge to pee I must go or I will pee myself.

Nurse: (turns to doctor)

Nurse: Dr. Chen, Anita Ford is complaining of frequency and dysuria. And she reports suffering urge incontinence.

Doctor: Sally, could you do a urinalysis on her urine?

Nurse: Sure…*(After the test)* Dr. Chen, I've done the urinalysis. Mrs. Ford's urine is positive for white blood cell, protein and occult blood.

Doctor: What colour is her urine?

Nurse: It's light red.

Doctor: It seems that she has a UTI (urinary tract infection, or urinary infection). Can you take a midstream urine (MSU) for her?

Nurse: Okay.

C. Stool (Feces) Report

Nurse: (turns to patient)

Nurse: Mr. Nelson, have you noticed any blood in your stool?

Patient: Yes. Every time I go, there is a little red blood that comes out with the poop.

Nurse: Have your stools been hard, normal, soft, watery or fatty?

Patient: They have been soft or watery.

Nurse: (turns to doctor)

Nurse: Dr. Lee, Mr. Nelson reports having small amount of blood in his stool. His stool has been loosely formed.

Doctor: Could you please test his stool?

Nurse: Sure…*(After the test)* His stool is positive for white blood cell, red blood cell and occult blood.

Unit 5

Lead-in

Listen and repeat.

Listen to the following sentences and repeat them. Pay attention to the pronunciation and intonation.

1. How strong is the pain?

2. What's the pain in your shoulder like?

3. When does the pain start/stop?

4. I've brought a pain chart so you can explain your pain a bit better.

5. Does anything make them worse?

6. What makes the pain better?

7. Do you feel anything else wrong when it's there?

8. What does the pain feel like?

9. How often do you get the pain?

10. Can you tell me on a scale of zero to ten what is the worst pain you've had in the last twenty-four hours in each area?

Task 1 Pronounce the words.

Write down the words according to the phonetic symbols below. And then listen and check.

1. aching   2. stabbing   3. sharp   4. tingling

5. burning   6. throbbing   7. tender   8. shooting

9. dull   10. colicky

Listen and practice.

Look at the pictures of people in pain. Listen to six short conversations (1-6) and match the pictures(a-f) to the conversations.

Conversation 1

Nurse: How are you feeling?

Patient: Not great. Can I have some painkillers, please?

Nurse: Sure. Where does it hurt?

Patient: My lower back's really aching.

Nurse: OK, I'll get the tablets and a heat pack, too.

Conversation 2

Nurse: Are you all right, Mrs. Jane?

Patient: No, I've got a really burning stomachache?

Nurse: Lie down on the bed and I'll get you some pain relief.

Patient: Thanks.

Conversation 3

Nurse: How do you feel this morning?

Patient: Awful, I've been having some throbbing pain in my head.

Nurse: Sit down on the bed and I'll run some tests.

Patient: Thanks.

Conversation 4

Nurse: Are you feeling better today?

Patient: Not really, I've got a bit of cram pain in my leg.

Nurse: OK, I'll get some heat pack for you.

Patient: Thanks.

Conversation 5

Nurse: Where don't you feel well, Daniel?

Patient: Well, I was knocked down by a car and when I got up, I had a stabbing pain in my rib.

Nurse: OK, relax. The doctor will examine you right now.

Patient: Thanks.

Conversation 6

Nurse: What has brought you here, Brian?

Patient: I cut my finger when cooking. I felt awful pain.

Nurse: OK, I'll take care of your wound. Don't worry.

Patient: Thanks.

Task 3 **Work in pairs.**

Listen to ten patients describing their pain, find out what kind of pain it is and where the pain is and fill in the table below. Practice describing pain to the medical staff according to the examples as below.

1. Every day I have trouble brushing my teeth because of **aching** pain in my arms.

2. Sometimes I have trouble standing up due to the **stabbing** pain in my backside.

3. Suddenly I felt a **sharp** pain in my back when I leaned forward to the ground to pick up the pen.

4. I frequently experience **tingling** pain in my extremities even when I don't do anything.

5. Every night I have trouble sleeping due to the **burning** pain in my stomach.

6. For over a month now, I've had an infrequent **throbbing pain** & pressure on the right side of my head.

7. Sometimes, I feel **tender** pain in my tummy.

8. I have had a **shooting** pain on the right side of my lower abdomen for the last 6 weeks or so.

9. Last night, I had a **dull** pain in the chest.

10. I suffered from **colicky** pain in my abdomen after I had an ice-cream.

Task 5 **Listen and practice.**

Listen to the conversation and fill in the blanks on the Pain Assessment Chart.

Nurse: Hello, John. My name is Jenny. I'm taking care of you today.

Patient: Hello, Jenny. Nice to meet you.

Nurse: How do you feel today?

Patient: I'm not very well today. I've got a lot of pain.

Nurse: Oh, dear, I'm sorry to hear that. I've brought a pain chart so you can explain your pain a bit better.

Patient: Er, it's fine.

Nurse: Where's the pain, John?

Patient: There are three areas which hurt.

Nurse: OK. Can you tell me on a scale of zero to ten what is the worst pain you've had in the last twenty-four hours in each area?

Patient: OK.

Nurse: Can you show me the first one on the picture of the body?

Patient: It's my left shoulder.

Nurse: OK. What's the pain in your shoulder like?

Patient: It's sharp pain, not throbbing pain.

Nurse: What sets the pain off?

Patient: It starts when I move or try to get out of bed.

Nurse: How strong is the pain right now?

Patient: Er, a five. I had to get back to bed because of the pain.

Nurse: OK, I'll label that pain "A". What makes the pain better?

Patient: The painkillers help and heat packs are good, too.

Nurse: OK. What about the next one?

Patient: The ulcer in the right leg.

Nurse: OK. That's "B". What starts the pain in your right leg?

Patient: It only hurts when the nurse changes the dressing.

Nurse: What's the pain like?

Patient: It's burning pain—around a four out of ten.

Nurse: What helps the pain?

Patient: Those non-stick dressings are good. And I have some pain relievers before the nurse does the dressing.

Nurse: OK. What about the last area of pain?

Patient: My lower back. It is the worst pain.

Nurse: Mm, it's where the main cancer is, isn't it?

Patient: Yes, my back aches a lot.

Nurse: I'll label that pain "C". How bad is the pain now?

Patient: It's nine at the moment.

Nurse: What makes the pain worse?

Patient: When I move or sit in the chair.

Nurse: Does the painkiller help?

Patient: A little but not much.

Nurse: That's not good, is it? I'll inform the doctor to check the orders for you.

Patient: Thanks. I might need some stronger medication.

Task 7 Pronounce the words.

Write down the words according to the phonetic symbols below. And then listen and check.

1. acupuncture
2. hypnotherapy
3. massage
4. aromatherapy
5. analgesia
6. hydrotherapy
7. heat pack
8. music therapy
9. chiropractic therapy
10. herbal therapy

Task 8 Listen and match.

Some patients choose to use complementary and alternative medicine (CAM) to treat their pain. Look at pictures below. Then listen to the audio about different examples of CAM (1-6) and match the pictures to the types of pain relief (a-f).

Example 1

The doctor administers some medication which can stop pain and which is taken by mouth or by injection.

Example 2

The therapist uses a heat pad which soothes some muscles.

Example 3

The therapists talk to the patient when he or she is "asleep" to influence their feelings about pain.

Example 4

This therapy uses natural oils to help control pain.

Example 5

Therapists rub or press parts of the body to relieve pain.

Example 6

The therapist uses fine needles to relieve pain.

Unit 6

Lead-in

Listen and repeat.

Listen to the following sentences and repeat them. Pay attention to the pronunciation and intonation.

1. Sally Taylor needs to take 10 milligrams of Zocor once a day by mouth, at bedtime for 90 days.
2. I've got your discharge medication here, Derrick. I just need to explain a few things to you.
3. This one is your antibiotic. Make sure you take it on an empty stomach.
4. The last one is the lotion for your rash. It's important that you shake the bottle so you mix the contents well.
5. Here are the eye drops. They only last a month so remember to discard the contents after this date.
6. Crosscheck the name of the medication on the Prescription Chart and the medication label.
7. I'm going to follow the "five rights" of medication administration for patient safety.
8. Yes, that's the correct drug, but it should have been ordered by its generic name, furosemide, not its brand name, Lasix.
9. I don't have the right to administer medication without a clear order.
10. Can you see the label to check the dose?

Task 1 Pronounce the words.

Work in pairs, match words in the box to pictures A-K. And read after the audio.

capsule; ointment; solution; suppository; powder; tablet; inhaler; syrup; spray; drop; injection

Task 3 Listen and complete.

In pairs, read the prescription and write them out in words. Then listen and check your answer. Practice explaining orders in turns.

1. Sally Taylor needs to take 10 milligrams of Zocor once a day by mouth, at bedtime for 90 days.
2. Diovan is for your blood pressure. Edna Cuthbert needs to take 40 milligrams of Diovan three times a day by mouth, before meals/after meals for 30 days.
3. Masoud Khan needs to take 20 milligrams of Fluvastatin twice a day by mouth for 7 days.

Task 5 Listen and practice.

Listen to two conversations between nurses and patients. Complete the following extracts from the conversations.

Conversation 1

Nurse: I've got your discharge medication here, Derrick. I just need to explain a few things to you.

Patient: Ok. What have you got there?

Nurse: This one is your antibiotic. Make sure you take it on an empty stomach.

Patient: Oh right. Take it before I eat?

Nurse: That's right. But if you feel upset in your stomach, you should let your doctor know. Now, this is your inhaler. You must rinse your mouth with water after you use it.

Patient: OK. Clean my mouth after I use it.

Nurse: Mm hm. The last one is the lotion for your rash. It's important that you shake the bottle so you mix the contents well.

Patient: OK, I'll do that.

Conversation 2

Nurse: Abby, your medications have come up from the pharmacy.

Patient: Oh good. I am waiting for them.

Nurse: Well, I've got two medications. Here are the eye drops. They only last a month so remember to discard the contents after this date.

Patient: OK. After September the 16th, I see.

Nurse: Don't forget to keep the eye drops in the fridge.

Patient: Oh, yes. Thanks for reminding me.

Nurse: You've also got a tablet to take twice a day. You must avoid too much sun with these tablets. They could burn easily.

Patient: Oh, OK.

Task 6 **Work in pairs.**

Practice giving precautions about medications according to your professional knowledge. Use the medication labels in task 4 and the phrases in the box below. And then listen to the audio and repeat.

1. Don't forget to keep the insulin in the fridge.

2. It's important that you shake the bottle before taking syrup.

3. Make sure you take antibiotics on an empty stomach.

4. Remember to rinse your mouth with water after you use inhaler.

5. You must complete the course of medication to get the optimised effect.

Task 8 **Listen and practice.**

Jenny, a Student Nurse, is doing a medication check with Joan, a Registered Nurse. Listen to the conversation and mark the order in which Jenny checks the five rights.

Joan: Hi, Jenny. Are you ready to go through this medication administration with me?

Jenny: Fine, OK.

Joan: All right. Here we are. Hello, Mrs. Gilbert. Do you mind if Jenny gives you your medications?

Mrs. Gilbert: No, dear, I don't mind at all.

Jenny: Thanks, Mrs. Gilbert. OK, I'm going to follow the "five rights" of medication administration for your safety. Mrs. Gilbert is ordered to have Lasix. Erm, it's on the tray as furosemide.

Joan: Yes, that's the correct drug, but it should have been ordered by its generic name, furosemide, not its brand name, Lasix.

Jenny: Yes, it can be unclear sometimes, can't it? Um, the medication is prescribed for Mrs. Eileen Gilbert, I'll just check the order on the chart. And Mrs. Gilbert, if you don't mind, I'd like to check your identity bracelet, too.

Mrs. Gilbert: Why would you do that? You know who I am.

Jenny: You'd be surprised, Mrs. Gilbert. Sometimes two patients with the same name are in the hospital at the same time.

Mrs. Gilbert: That can be so, right?

Joan: Right. What route of administration do you have to use?

Jenny: Oral, I think. The doctor hasn't written that in it.

Joan: That's a problem, isn't it? The doctor may want to use the oral route or IV route?

Jenny: Ah, I see what you mean.

Joan: What about the dose?

Jenny: It's not on the chart. It's usually 40mg, but the dose would depend on her conditions.

Joan: Quite right. You couldn't assume it. It could lead to dangerous consequences.

Jenny: Mm, there's a problem with frequency and time of administration as well. The doctor hasn't noted down the frequency at which the medication is to be given or the times. That's a problem. I mustn't administer medication without a clear order.

Joan: Well done. Now, tell me. Is it all right to administer medication to Mrs. Gilbert?

…

Unit 7

Lead-in

Listen and repeat.

Listen to the following sentences and repeat them. Pay attention to the pronunciation and intonation.

1. The cannula hurts a lot and the IV's not dripping any more.

2. You've still got six doses of IV antibiotics so we need to put a new line.

3. Every time you lifted your arm the infusion stopped.

4. It means inflammation of the vein. More often than not it's caused by a nosocomial infection of staph, originating in hospital.

5. That's why we check the cannula site and take the cannula out at the first sign of infection.

6. She's got an eight hourly litre of normal saline up.

7. Here is her hospital label … Mabyn Hadfield … unit number 62388 … date of birth 12th January, 1920.

8. One litre of normal saline over eight hours.

9. The date is 30th of May, the route is IV and the fluid is five percent Dextrose.

10. The rate is one litre over ten hours. That's easy to work out. One litre—a thousand mils—divided by ten hours.

Task 2 **Recognize and read.**

Label the IV equipment (1-6) below using the words in the box. Then read the terms correctly with the audio.

1. IV pole
2. IV solution
3. IV line
4. IV infusion pump
5. IV cannula
6. fluid balance chart

Task 3 **Read aloud and check.**

Read the following notes and put a tick (√) in the correct column. And then listen to the audio and check.

1. a thousand
2. at eleven millilitres, on the thirtieth of May
3. five hundred millilitres an hour
4. one hundred and sixty-seven drops per minute
5. five percent
6. normal saline

Task 4 **Work in pairs.**

Put these words in order to make sentences. Listen and check your answers.

1. Check the IV solution against the physician's orders.
2. Wash hands thoroughly before inserting an IV.
3. Use sterile technique when inserting an IV line.
4. Prime the IV tubing to remove air from the system.
5. Label the tubing, and solution bags clearly, indicating the date and time when changed.

Task 5 **Role-play.**

Listen to the conversation between the nurse and the patient and then play the roles.

N: Good morning, Ms. Smith. It's time to give you intravenous infusion.

P: Excuse me, could you tell me about the use of the intravenous fluid?

N: Of course. The fluid can provide energy for you and prevent you from electrolytic imbalances after the operation.

(*IV infusion is set up.*)

P: Would you please let the fluid drop more quickly?

N: Your intravenous fluid must be given slowly so as not to overload you.

P: Is it possible for my sister to stay here with me?

N: Yes, of course. But I don't think it is necessary. Your condition isn't that serious.

P: Oh, I see.

N: Is there anything I can do for you?

P: I feel a little cold. Could you help me adjust the air conditioner?

N: Please wait a moment. Do you want another blanket?

P: No, thanks.

N: Just press the button if you need any help.

P: Thank you. Sorry to bother you.

N: You are welcome.

Task 6 **Listen and match.**

Listen to the audio and match the medical terms to their meanings, and then act out the dialogue.

N: Hello. Mrs. Smith. Can I just check that your IV cannula is all right before I put up the next infusion?

P: Oh, thanks. I was just going to buzz you. The cannula hurts a lot and the IV's not dripping any more.

N: OK, it sounds like an infiltration. It occurs when the fluid leaks into the tissues and doesn't drip into the vein. I'd also like to check why it hurts. Can I have a look? Hm, it's quite warm, isn't it?

P: Yes, and it looks red, too.

N: So you've got warmth, erythema—that's the redness—and the tenderness.

P: Yes, it started being sore a little while ago.

N: Sounds like an infection. I'll have a look on your Care Plan to see when the doctor put the IV in. Hm … three days ago. OK, well, it'll need to be resited anyway.

P: What do you mean?

N: It means that I'll call the doctor to come and put in a new one. I'll stop this drip now and take out your cannula.

P: I thought that's what you'd have to do. Why do I still have to have one? Can't they leave the cannula out?

N: Sorry, you've still got six doses of IV antibiotics so we need to put in a new line.

P: Right, OK. I hope they can find a more convenient spot to put it in.

N: I know it was a nuisance, and it was positional, too. Every time you lifted your arm the infusion stopped. The thing is that there is a lower risk of phlebitis if we put the cannula in your hand.

P: Phlebitis? Is that infection?

N: Yes. It means inflammation of the vein. More often than not it's caused by a nosocomial infection of staph, or staphylococci bacteria originating in hospital. Staph is usually found on the hands. The best way to prevent infection entering is for health workers to wash their hands properly before touching the cannula site and to use aseptic technique when putting in a new cannula.

P: I see.

N: That's why we check the cannula site and take the cannula out at the first sign of infection. Our hospital follows Evidence-Based Practice guidelines which suggest that we take IV cannula out after seventy-two hours and that we change the IV giving sets at the same time. The number of days the IV is kept is recorded in the Care Plan.

Task 7 **Listen and complete.**

Listen to the audio and complete the chart.

(A= Alicia, ward nurse; K= Kimber, ward nurse.)

A: Kimber, I'm just off to lunch. Do you mind keeping an eye on Miss Clarke's fluids?

K: Sure, no problem. When did she have the IV put in?

A: On admission yesterday. It was just to KVO while she was having her IV antibiotics, but she became dehydrated and still wasn't drinking much. That's why they had to increase her fluids.

K: She was in a bad way when she came in, wasn't she? What's up now?

A: She's got an eight hourly litre of normal saline, but it's just through. Do you mind checking out another bag with me? I can go to lunch then.

K: Sure. Have you got the prescription chart with you?

A: Yeah, here it is. Here is her hospital label ... Mabyn Clarke ... unit number 62388 ... date of birth 21st January 1980.

K: OK. normal saline—that's the litre up to now?

A: That's right. One litre of normal saline over eight hours. It went up at 3:00 hours and it's through now at 11: 00 so I'll write that in here. And I'll write the amount of a thousand millilitres. Now we can check out the next one. The date is the 30th of May, the route is IV and the fluid is five percent Dextrose.

K: 30th, yes, IV, yes, five percent Dextrose, yes.

A: OK. We can check the IV infusion now. Here is the bag. I'll just show you. Five percent Dextrose. It expires on the sixteenth of July 2020. Can you see the expiry date on the bag is OK?

K: Yeah, five percent Dextrose, expires on the sixteenth of July 2020. Correct.

A: Right, so let me write it in. 30th May, 11: 00. The rate is one litre over ten hours. That's easy to work out. One litre—a thousand millilitres—divided by ten hours. That's a hundred millilitres an hour.

K: Looks good.

A: OK. My initial here under Nurse one. A.C.

K: And my initial here under Nurse two. K.B.

A: Thanks. Do you mind putting it up so I can have my break now?

K: No, go ahead. I'll put it up for you.

A: Thanks.

Task 8 **Listen and complete.**

Listen to the audio and circle the details you hear in the chart.

(K=Kasia, the ward nurse; H=Harris, the surgical registrar.)

K: Good morning, Ward 7 West, Kasia speaking.

H: Hello, it's Dr. Harris here. I'm the surgical registrar for your ward. I was bleeped about resiting an IV cannula for Mrs. Blake. Can I speak to the nurse looking after her?

K: Oh, Michael's looking after Mrs. Blake today. He's just on a break. Can I take a message for him?

H: Yeah. Could you please ask Michael to call me and let me know how quickly the cannula needs to be resited? … um, let me know when Mrs. Blake's next IV antibiotics are due.

K: OK. Let me just read that message back to you. You want Michael to call and tell you when the cannula needs to be resited and when the next IV antibiotics are due?

H: That's right.

K: OK. I'll make sure I pass your message on to Michael. He'll be back from his break in about five minutes or so. Er, can I get a contact number so Michael can return your call?

H: Sure, my bleeper number is 467. Thanks, Kasia.

K: You are welcome.

Unit 8

Lead-in

Listen and repeat.

Listen to the following sentences and repeat them. Pay attention to the pronunciation and intonation.

1. Would you like some help to wash?
2. I can help you to wash now, if you're ready.
3. Would you like me to give you a hand to shave?
4. Could you please change my sheets? I'm sorry but I've wetted the bed.
5. Would you please make beds from five to ten?
6. Would you prefer a shower or a bed sponge?
7. I'll just get the commode chair and then I can take you down to the bathroom.
8. Could you please tend to David White's mouth and eye care?
9. I'm just going to clean your mouth with these swabs which have been dipped in mouthwash, OK?
10. I'm just going to use cotton buds soaked with saline to clean the lower part of your nostrils out. We won't go in too far.

Task 1 Work in pairs.

Label the pictures with the words in the box, and listen and check. Then describe the function of each object.

1. washbasin	2. towel	3. toothbrush	4. gloves
5. brush	6. shampoo	7. detergent	8. clinical disposable bag
9. sink	10. toothpaste	11. bucket	12. razor
13. kidney basin	14. shaving cream	15. pyjamas	16. paper towels
17. blanket	18. bin	19. swab	20. soap

Task 2 Pronounce the words.

Write down the words according to the phonetic symbols below. And then listen and check.

1. inspection	2. hygiene	3. spillage	4. fluid	5. urine
6. staff	7. considerate	8. swab	9. sponge	10. mouthwash

Task 3 **Listen and complete.**

Listen to a short dialogue between a hospital administrator and a ward cleaner. Complete the hygiene report below by filling in the missing words.

(A=administrator; L=Linda, ward cleaner)

A:　　　　Hi, Linda! I have something important to tell you.

L:　　　　Oh? What is it?

A:　　　　Well, I have to talk to you about the hygiene inspection.

L:　　　　OK. How was the score?

A:　　　　Em. 2 out of 10.

L:　　　　Oh really? Well, they came at a very bad time, you know, nearly 12 o'clock…

A:　　　　Mmm. And I have the report here. Let's see the important things… Under "Ward Hygiene", Look! Door handles are not regularly cleaned, and beds are not always cleaned between patients…

L:　　　　Oh, sorry.

A:　　　　Toilets must be cleaned every three hours a day but they are only cleaned twice a day.

L:　　　　Ah…

A:　　　　Floors must be cleaned every two hours a day but they are only cleaned once a day. And under "Spillages of Bodily Fluids" the report says that the average time was 30 minutes to clean up a spill of urine. And it says nurses' knowledge of MRSA is good, but…

L:　　　　They always wear gloves…

A (cuts in): Not good enough. Look, it says here, nurses must wash hands before putting on gloves and after removing gloves. But they didn't wash hands after taking off gloves.

L:　　　　Well, we certainly need to improve, but you know we are really very short-staffed.

A:　　　　Well, emm, I'll see to it soon.

L:　　　　Thank you! You're so considerate!

Task 4 **Listen and complete.**

Listen to a lecture about personal hygiene care and take notes by answering the following questions and completing the sentences. Then practice the dialogue in pairs.

Bathing The primary purpose of bathing is to cleanse the body of all dirt, sweat, germs and other things. This cleansing protects our first-level defense against infection, and it also promotes good circulation and patient comfort.

There are three different types of baths: a complete bed bath, a partial bath, and a tub or shower bath. With all types of baths, the water temperature must be safe. A shower chair, tub chair, grab bars, a nonskid bath or shower mat are also very important to prevent accidents. When patients prefer a shower or tub bath rather than a bed bath, they will often need assistance getting in and out of the shower or tub to prevent a fall or an injury.

Perineal Care Perineal care, like the bathing of the skin, prevents infections, odors and irritation in that area. Perineal care is done with the bed bath, shower or tub bath and it is done more often for patients affected with incontinence and diaphoresis.

Shaving Male patients often want a facial shave once a day or once every couple of days; female patients usually want their underarms and legs shaved about once a week.

Oral Hygiene Oral hygiene is done at least twice a day and more often as needed. Oral hygiene consists of brushing the teeth, flossing the teeth, and rinsing the mouth. Partial and full dentures are also brushed and rinsed.

Foot Care Feet are washed with bath and more often as needed. Diabetics and other patients at risk for infections should get special foot and toe nail care and monitoring. For example, the feet must be completely cleaned and dried and examined daily for any sign of skin breakdown, corns, bleeding, broken, chipped or absent nails, as well as blue or pale nail beds.

Hair Care Patients' hair can be washed with shampoo and conditioner in the shower, bathtub and in bed with a special bed tray or dry shampoo. Patients should also be encouraged to comb or brush their hair a couple of times a day.

Nail Care Patients' nail care is another important area of hygiene and patients' nails need to be checked daily, to observe them for any irregularities. The patients' nails should appear clean, because dirt can cause infection, and jagged nails may cause injuries to the patients or to the staff attending to them.

Task 5 **Work in pairs.**

Listen to the dialogue between a patient and a nurse about the morning care. Answer the related questions and then practice in pairs.

(Every morning before the patients wake up, the nurses must get everything ready to carry out different kinds of nursing duties for the patients. The following dialogue happened during a nurse's morning care.)

(N=nurse; P=patient)

N: Good morning. Did you sleep well last night?

P: Good morning. I slept very well.

N: Would you like me to bring you a bedpan?

P: Yes, please.

N: Let me help you to clean up.

P: OK. Thanks a lot.

N: Here is some water, your toothbrush and toothpaste.

P: But I've got a pain in my mouth.

N: Don't worry. I'll have a look after you finish brushing your teeth.

(*After the examination*)

N: There are some small ulcers.

P: Are they serious?

N: Not really. Since you cannot move easily yourself, I'll help you to clean up and make you feel comfortable.

P: Thank you.

N: Let me fluff up your pillow.

P: That's nice.

N: Please turn over to the other side. I'll rub your back with a hot towel and then massage it.

P: What's it for?

N: Well, it is mainly to stimulate your blood circulation to prevent bedsores.

P: Oh, I see. And my clothes are all wet from sweating during the night. Would you please change them for me?

N: Surely. I've already brought clean and dry ones for you. I'll help you to change.

P: It's very nice of you.

N: And I'll also be changing your bed sheets.

P: Good. Must I get out of bed?

N: No, you needn't. I can do the change without your getting out of bed. You just lie in bed and I can do everything for you.

P: All right. Thank you.

N: My pleasure.

Task 6 Work in pairs.

Listen to a recording and complete the table below. Discuss in pairs what a nurse usually does when tending to morning and evening care.

After breakfast, the nurse usually offers assistance with morning care, including toileting, oral care, bathing, back massage, skin care measures (e.g. for to prevent pressure ulcer), hair care, dressing, and positioning for comfort, etc. Morning care is often characterized as self-care, partial care, and complete care. Self-care patients are capable of managing their personal hygiene independently. These patients should be offered a back massage. Partial care patients always receive morning hygiene care at the bedside or seated near the sink in the bathroom. Because of weakness, these patients may be able to wash only parts of their bodies that are within easy reach. The nurse washes the back and legs because these body parts have the most secretions and are difficult to reach. Complete care patients require nursing assistance with all aspects of personal hygiene. A complete bed bath is done or the patient is taken to the shower or tub.

Before the patients go to bed in the evening, the nurse again offers assistance with toileting, washing of face and hands, and oral care. Many patients find a back massage helps them to relax and fall asleep and this should be offered routinely. Soiled bed linens or clothing should be changed and the patient should be positioned comfortably. Make sure that there are no items, which the patient could slip on, or fall over, such as chairs or linens, on the floor. The call light and any other objects the patients need (e.g. urinal, radio, or water glass) should be within easy reach.

Task 7 Work in pairs.

Particular attention should be paid to the areas of bony prominences which are at a high risk for pressure ulcers. Listen and write out the Chinese meaning of each word according to the picture below.

1. occiput   2. scapula   3. elbow   4. sacrum

5. heel	6. toes	7. thigh	8. trochanter femur
9. lower leg	10. upper humerus	11. rib cage	12. patella

Task 8 Listen and complete.

Listen to the following recordings on prevention and treatment of pressure ulcers and complete the table by filling in the missing words. Then discuss in pairs.

If you are caring for someone confined to a bed or chair for any period of time, it's important to be aware of the risk of pressure ulcers. To prevent skin damage, you need to relieve the pressure, reduce the time that pressure is applied and improve skin quality. There are some ways to prevent pressure ulcers such as position changes, daily skin care, a nutritious diet and lifestyle changes and so on.

Position changes to prevent pressure ulcers

Patients who use a wheelchair are advised to shift position within their chair about every 15 minutes. People who spend most of their time in bed are advised to change positions at least once every two hours, even during the night, and to avoid lying directly on their hipbones.

Daily skin care to prevent pressure ulcers

Check the skin at least daily for redness or signs of discoloration.

Keep the skin at the right moisture level, as damage is more likely to occur if the skin is the either too dry or too moist.

Never massage bony areas because the skin is too delicate.

Diet and lifestyle changes to avoid pressure ulcers

Make sure the patient eats a healthy and nutritious diet.

Be aware of using good hygiene practices.

Maintain appropriate activity levels.

Make sure the patient quits smoking.

Treatment for pressure ulcers

There is a variety of treatments to manage pressure ulcers and promote healing, depending on the severity of the pressure ulcers. The strategies include:

regular position changes

special mattresses and beds that reduce pressure

dressings to keep the ulcers moist and the surrounding skin dry

regular cleaning with appropriate solutions, depending on what stage the ulcers are at

specific drugs and chemicals applied to the area, if an infection persists

surgery to remove the damaged tissues

operations to close the wound, using skin grafts if necessary

continuing supportive lifestyle habits such as eating a healthy and nutritious diet.

Task 9 Listen and speak.

Listen to a sample dialogue and then make a new dialogue on your own. Pay attention to the pronunciation and intonation while listening and imitating. Work in pairs, practise speaking and performing the dialogue.

Nurse: Liu Feng, you're welcome to practise here. Now let's go to see Mrs. Brown.

Liu Feng: OK. It seems she's unconscious.

Nurse: Yeah. She is.

Liu Feng: I was taught that the care of an unconscious patient would be a comprehensive one and almost cover all the basic nursing skills.

Nurse: You're quite right. Today we'll just focus on the hygienic care for the patient.

Liu Feng: Personal hygiene usually includes skin care, bathing and the care of mouth, eyes, ears and nose.

Nurse: You get the point. We do oral hygiene twice a day. We use a cotton stick to brush the patient's teeth and mucous membranes, especially the lips. They're easy to get dry and have debris because the unconscious patient often uses the mouth to breathe.

Liu Feng: How do you care for the eyes, ears or nose?

Nurse: Use eye drops, eye ointment, or eye patches to prevent infection. This patient has tubes in her nostrils, so it is essential to lubricate them regularly.

Liu Feng: I see.

Nurse: Skin is the first defence against infections, so we should maintain the patient's skin integrity. Each time after a bed bath, we should dry the patient thoroughly and massage her.

Liu Feng: It can stimulate the blood circulation and prevent bedsores.

Nurse: Right. Do you know what places are prone to bedsores?

Liu Feng: Bone prominences, such as occiput, neck, shoulder, elbow, pelvis and heel, etc. They're usually under pressure so that the blood circulation is poor.

Nurse: In addition to massage, we should turn the patient every 2 hours to relieve pressure. Remember to change bed linens whenever they're wet. Do not drag the patient when moving her.

Liu Feng: There're so many things to learn. I'll keep them in mind.

Unit 9

Lead-in

Listen and repeat.

Listen to the following sentences and repeat them. Pay attention to the pronunciation and intonation.

1. How has your appetite been lately?

2. Do you feel sick or uncomfortable in any way?

3. I can really understand that you don't feel too hungry with all your discomfort at present, but your body needs the nutrition so that you can regain your strength and energy.

4. Please let us know if there is something you particularly feel like eating.

5. How much food do you normally eat in a day?

6. How big would each meal be?

7. Have you noticed experiencing any weight gain or weight loss lately?

8. The patient is a healthy weight/slightly underweight/obese for her height.

9. How would you describe your diet?

10. What kinds of food does your diet mostly consist of?

Task 2 Pronounce the words.

Write down the words according to the phonetic symbols below. And then listen and check.

1. sugar	2. protein	3. dairy	4. fats	5. health
6. vitamin	7. mineral	8. energy	9. calcium	10. carbohydrate

Task 4 Listen and complete.

Listen to the dialogue and complete the Nursing Assessment Form and the following sentences. And then practice the dialogue with your partner.

(N=nurse; S=Steven, patient)

N: What's your normal weight, Steven?

S: I'm about sixty-six kilos, I guess.

N: I see my colleague weighed you earlier and you're currently around fifty-three kilos. OK, and how tall are you?

S: About one metre seventy-two.

N: Mmm, that gives you a BMI around seventeen point nine. What weight would you like to be?

S: The same as before, sixty-six.

N: I just need to ask you a few questions, if I may. Erm, do you have any food allergies we should know about?

S: Yes, I'm allergic to peanuts.

N: That's important for us to know, thanks. Anything else? What about lactose intolerance?

S: I'm sorry?

N: Dairy products. Do you have any problems digesting dairy products, like milk?

S: No, no, I can drink milk. I don't like cheese though.

N: OK. When was your last meal?

A: About ten, last night, when I finished work. A bowl of soup, some toast…

Task 5 Work in pairs.

Put these words in order to make sentences. Listen and check your answer.

1. What kind of diet do you recommend for me?

2. Some patients find it helpful to eat small meals five or six times a day.

3. How has your appetite been lately?

4. Your body needs the nutrition so that you can regain your strength and energy.

5. Excess weight is associated with an increased risk of heart disease.

6. You should avoid fatty meat and fried foods in order to prevent high blood cholesterol.

Task 6 Role-play.

Listen to the recording and play the role.

(N=nurse; P=patient)

N: Would you mind telling me what your weight is?

P: Two hundred and eleven pounds.

N: Your height, please?

P: I'm five feet six inches tall. How severe is my weight problem?

N: Generally, a patient with a body mass index, or BMI (Body Mass Index) of 25 to 29.9 is considered overweight; one with a BMI of 30 or higher is considered obese. And yours is 34.1. I'm afraid it's a little serious.

P: Without intervention, what should I expect?

N: Excess weight is associated with an increased risk of heart disease, stroke, high blood pressure, diabetes, gallstones and some forms of cancer.

P: How much weight should I lose?

N: Permanent weight loss is extraordinarily difficult, studies show, and ideal weights are rarely reached. A weight loss goal should be realistic, researchers say, and you should also take into account your family history and current risk factors. Many people find it useful to set goals in stages — for example, to lose 10 pounds within two months, then another 10, and so forth.

P: What kind of diet do you recommend for me?

N: Avoid diets that exclude the entire categories of food. Popular high-protein menus may work for some patients in the short term, some researchers have found, but fruits and vegetables should be the foundation of any long-term diet.

P: Does meal frequency matter?

N: Some patients find it helpful to eat small meals five or six times a day. Complicated regimens involving macronutrients consumed only at certain time of the day have not been well supported by research.

P: Thank you for your advice.

Task 7 Listen and complete.

Complete the passage according to the recording, and then repeat it.

Diabetes is a disease that occurs when your blood glucose, also called blood sugar, is too high. Blood glucose is your main source of energy and comes from the food you eat. Insulin, a hormone made by the pancreas, helps glucose from food get into your cells to be used for energy. Sometimes your body doesn't make enough—or any—insulin or doesn't use insulin well. Glucose then stays in your blood and doesn't reach your cells.

Over time, having too much glucose in your blood can cause health problems. Although diabetes has no cure, you can take steps to manage your diabetes and stay healthy.

Sometimes people call diabetes "a touch of sugar" or "borderline diabetes". These terms suggest that someone doesn't really have diabetes or has a less serious case, but every case of diabetes is serious.

The most common types of diabetes are type 1, type 2, and gestational diabetes.

Task 8 Listen and choose the best answer.

Listen to the recording and then choose the best answer to each question.

(N=nurse; P=patient)

N: Why have you come to see the doctor?

P: I have had a bad headache for some time. They would often subside a little, but they have never healed completely.

N: Is there anything else that bothers you besides the headache?

P: I feel tired and itchy all over.

N: Have you lost weight recently?

P: I think I have.

N: How is your appetite?

P: I have a very good appetite, and I feel hungry all the time.

N: Do you drink lots of water and go to the toilet often?

P: Yes, I drink lots of water, but I still feel thirsty. And I have to go to the toilet often.

N: How long have you had these symptoms?

P: More than six months.

N: We'd like to take your urine and blood samples to check their sugar contents. Doctor Wang will see you soon. Please wait for a moment.

Task 9 Complete and practice.

Sample:

(N=nurse; P=patient)

(After the consultation)

P: Dr. Wang told me I have diabetes.

N: Yes, I know. Are there any members in your family who have diabetes?

P: Yes, my father has it.

N: Dr. Wang has ordered that you should follow a diabetic diet and insulin therapy. Here are instructions for your therapy, which by the way, you'll have to administer by yourself at home. We'll help you if you find it difficult. Here are some medicines for your headache.

P: Thank you very much. Could you tell me something about the diabetic diet?

N: As the doctor told you, you should stick to a special diet and avoid sugar and sweets.

P: What else should I know?

N: You'd better learn something about diabetes and have your blood and urine tested regularly. Please stick to your new diet, take your medicine regularly and do some exercises. I'm sure you will feel better soon.

P: Thank you for your advice.

Unit 10

Lead-in

Listen and repeat.

Listen to the following sentences and repeat them. Pay attention to the pronunciation and intonation.

1. We are going to do the operation on you tomorrow.
2. I'm afraid you'll have to be operated on for appendicitis.
3. We'll give you anesthesia.
4. If you feel any pain during the operation, just let me know.
5. Have you signed the consent yet?
6. I'd like to shave off the hair around the operation area.
7. I'll give you an enema tonight.
8. After that, please don't take any food or water before the operation.
9. The purpose of this is to make sure that you have an empty stomach when you have surgery.
10. Please remove all nail polish, gel or similar nails on both of the hands prior to the time of surgery.

Task 1 Pronounce the words.

Write down the words according to the phonetic symbols below. And then listen and check.

1. operation	2. signature	3. anaesthetist	4. antiseptic
5. interfere	6. fluid	7. muscle	8. enema

Task 2 & Task 3 Listen and complete.

Marie Wiseman, 45-year-old, is admitted for chronic appendicitis and ready for appendectomy. Nancy, the Ward Nurse, prepares Mrs. Wiseman for her operation by telling her about the pre-operative routine. Listen to the conversation and complete the following sentences.

(N=nurse; P=patient)

N: Hello, Mrs. Wiseman. I'm Nancy. I'll be looking after you today. Have you settled in yet?

P: Yes, dear. I've met all the ladies in my room. I just have to wait for the operation now, don't I?

N: Yes. I'm going to look at the operation list when it comes out later today so I can tell you where you are on the list. I just need to go through some pre-op things with you. Is that okay?

P: Yes, that's fine.

N: First, I'll check your consent form. Is that your signature?

P: Yes, dear. I signed it in the doctor's clinic before I came to the hospital.

N: Good. Now, I'll get you to take off your nail polish later today so the anaesthetist will be able to see your nail beds.

P: Oh, all right.

N: And you'll also need to shower with this antiseptic wash. Here's a sachet of the wash for you. Just wash all over using the antiseptic wash as you would with soap.

P: Okay, I'll do that tonight before I go to bed.

N: Great. I'll get you to have another shower with the antiseptic wash in the morning. I'll give you another sachet in a while.

P: Will my tummy be shaved before the operation?

N: No, it won't. We used to shave the operation area but the policy has changed now. If the area doesn't interfere with the surgery, then it isn't shaved.

P: Oh, that's good. I remember having it done many years ago when I had an operation. It wasn't very comfortable.

N: I know what you mean. Now, I'm going to order you clear fluids for today. That means you'll just be on liquids today. Then you'll be Nil By Mouth after midnight.

P: Does that mean I won't be able to eat or drink anything after midnight, will I?

N: No, you won't. The reason for this is that when you have an anaesthetic, your muscles relax. If you have anything in your stomach it could rise up into your throat and you might inhale it.

P: Oh, I see. I certainly don't want that to happen.

N: No, not at all. I'll get you to take a special bowel preparation drink later to clean out your bowel. You'll also need a small enema to help you to open your bowels. This is so that when the surgeon operates, there is less chance of contamination from the bowel contents.

P: It's quite a business, isn't it?

N: Yes, it does take a bit of preparation. Oh, I'm going to do one last thing. I'm gonna to get you some anti-embolic stockings. They're very firm stockings; you put them on to support your legs. You wear them to prevent deep vein thrombosis—DVTs—or clots in your veins.

P: That's all right then. They won't be too much of a bother, I'm sure.

Task 5 Listen and answer.

Mr. Kim, 50-year-old, is booked for tumour resection under gastroscope tomorrow. Listen to Nadia, the Ward Nurse, explaining what Mr. Kim can expect when he returns to the ward after his operation, and answer the following questions.

(N=nurse; P=patient)

N: Good morning, Mr. Kim. I'm Nadia. I'll be looking after you today.

P: Hi, Nadia. Nice to meet you.

N: Well, I want to have a talk with you about your operation tomorrow.

P: Oh, is everything all right? There's nothing wrong, is there?

N: No, no, not at all, everything's fine. I'll just want to go through what will happen when you come back to the ward after the operation. People always feel better when they know what to expect.

P: Oh, yes, you're right. I'm so nervous about the operation.

N: Oh, don't be that nervous. Just take it easy. I'll go through it all now, and you'll have the opportunity to ask any questions as you like.

P: Thanks. I feel silly being so worried. I'm not normally like this.

N: That's OK, Mr. Kim. It's quite normal to feel a bit apprehensive. Um, I'll try and cover everything so you're prepared for what'll happen after the operation. I see you've brought the leaflet about the keyhole surgery.

P: Yes, it was sent to me at home last week. The only thing I know is that I won't have a big cut so the operation won't leave a big scar.

N: That's right. Keyhole surgery is also called minimally invasive surgery because it's performed with the use of a gastroscope, using small incisions or surgical cuts. The surgeon passes the gastroscope through your throat and is able to see the inside of the stomach, then removes the tumour through the same tube. The surgeon won't puncture your tummy.

P: Will I feel the pain?

N: No, you don't need to worry about that. You'll have a general anaesthesia, so you won't feel anything during the surgery.

P: Shall I have a drip in my arm?

N: Yes, you shall. You'll come back with an IV and some fluids running, just until you can eat and drink again.

P: Will I be able to eat straight away?

N: You'll have had a tube down your throat for the anaesthetic, so we'll need to make sure that your swallow reflex is working again after the tube's been removed. We'll also need to be sure that your bowels are working again before you try eating small amounts of food.

P: Oh, is that why they do that? I never knew. It makes sense to go slowly.

N: The other tube you'll have is an indwelling catheter, which they'll put in while you are in the theatre. It can be taken out when you're back to the ward and think you can void again—um, I mean, pass urine. Well, you won't have the catheter for too long.

P: Er, I hope so.

Task 7 Listen and complete.

Angela, the Ward Nurse, is checking Natasha Slessor for a surgery. Listen to the conversation and complete the parts mentioned in the conversation of the Pre-operative Checklist. Tick in the appropriate boxes marked YES or NO or N/A (Not Applicable).

N: Hello, Natasha. I'll just go through this checklist with you, and then I'll give you a pre-medication to relax you a bit, OK? Feeling all right?

P: Yes, I think I'm OK. The evening nurse went through everything about the operation with me last night so I know what to expect.

N: Good. Now, first of all I'm going to verify who you are, including your hospital number. You'll be asked the same information by lots of people along the way. Don't worry. It's just our checking system. Ah, now, can you tell me your full name, please?

P: Sure. Natasha Slessor.

N: Can I check your identity bracelets, too, please?

P: Yes, here they are.

N: Thanks, Natasha. That's 2018414, er, that's correct. Can you tell me what operation you're going to have?

P: Oh, um, they're going to fix the ligament in my left ankle.

N: Right, so that's a left ankle arthroscopy for a ligament repair. Er, great. Have you signed a consent form for the operation?

P: Yes, I signed it yesterday.

N: I'll just show you this signature. Is this your signature?

P: Yes, that's my signature.

N: OK, now did the surgeon come up and mark the operation site?

P: Yes, look, I've got the pen marks on my left ankle.

N: Yes, you have. Right, now I've got all your charts together—um, Drug Chart, Prescription Chart for IV fluids, Patient Record and Fluid Balance Chart. So, I'll tick that section. Um, have you had any X-rays done in the hospital?

P: Yes, I had an X-ray when I first came in.

N: Right, I'll get them and add them to your chart, which we'll take down to the Theatre. Do you have any allergies?

P: Er, no, not that I know of.

N: OK, that's a "No" for allergies. And, er, I'll circle "No" next to "Red bracelet worn" as you don't need one. Now, on to your teeth. Do you have any caps on your teeth, or crowns, or bridges?

P: No, I don't.

N: OK, I can write "No" for that, too. You don't have dentures either, do you?

P: No, all my own teeth.

N: Yeah, I thought so, but we have to ask to be sure. The operation site wasn't shaved, was it?

P: No, the surgeon just came and marked the operation area.

N: Right. Er, have you taken off your nail polish?

P: Yes, I did that this morning. Why do I have to take if off?

N: It's to minimize the infection and also to make it easier to check your circulation while you're under anaesthetic. Um, I need you to take off any jewellery you have. Metal is also a safety risk in the Theatre.

P: Oh, I didn't bring any jewellery to the hospital, but I don't really want to take my wedding ring off.

N: That's all right. I'll just tape it on securely so that the metal can be covered.

P: Thanks.

N: OK. Next question. Do you have any piercings?

P: No, I don't.

N: Right, so that's also "N/A" for piercings—it's not applicable to you. I've nearly finished the questions. How are you doing? Can I keep going?

P: Yes, I'm OK. I feel quite relaxed.

N: Right, I can see you've got a theatre gown on. Have you got your anti-embolic stockings on?

P: Yes, here they are, on nicely and smoothly as you showed me. I've even put on the disposable knickers you left me.

N: Good work. Er, ah, when was the last time you passed urine?

P: About five minutes before you came to check me. So, ten twenty I think.

N: OK, the last void was 10: 20 a.m. Let me see, I need to circle N/A next to catheterized because you don't have a catheter. Now, when was the last time you had something to eat or drink?

P: Er, I had dinner last night at 6 p.m., I think, and a last drink of water at 11 p.m. before the nurse put up the Nil By Mouth sign and took the water jug away.

N: That's good. As long as you have the last drink at least six hours before surgery, you don't want to risk vomiting after your surgery. All right, I'm going to give you your pre-medication now.

P: Er, pre-med? Does that mean I'm going to sleep now?

N: No, it's not an anaesthetic. You'll just feel calm and relaxed.

P: That's good.

N: There you are. Now, I'll just sign the checklist and we'll wait for the porters to take you to Theatres.

Task 8 & Task 9 Listen and complete.

Julia, the Theatre Nurse, checks the patient's details related to the operation. She uses the area in the column marked O/T (Operating Theatre). Listen to the conversation and tick the sections of the Checklist that Julia double-checks.
(J=Julia, theare nurse; P=patient)

J: Hello, I'm Julia. I'm a Theatre Nurse and I'm going to check you in today. How are you doing?

P: All right.

J: That's good. I'm just going to go through this Checklist again. OK? Um, I know you've already answered many of these questions, but we like to double-check everything, OK?

P: Yes, that's fine.

J: Right, can you tell me your full name, please?

P: Yes, Natasha Slessor.

J: Thank you. I'll have a quick look at your identification bracelet if I may?

P: Sure, here it is.

J: Natasha Slessor, number 2018414, correct. Can you tell me what operation you're having today?

P: Yes, I'm having the ligament in my left ankle repaired.

J: Mm, did you sign a consent form for the operation?

P: Yes, I did.

J: Is this your signature on the consent form?

P: Yes, it is.

J: All right, nearly finished. Have you had a pre-med?

P: Yes, I had an injection just before I came here.

J: Mm, pre-med given and signed for. Great. All right, I'll sign the Checklist and you've already got a theatre cap to cover your hair. You'll be waiting here for a few more minutes and then we'll take you through. Are you all right there?

P: Yes, thanks.

Unit 11

Lead-in

Listen and repeat.

Listen to the following sentences and repeat them. Pay attention to the pronunciation and intonation.

1. I've got David Smith back from the theatre.
2. I'll just go through the operation report with you.
3. I'm awake now, but I still feel a bit groggy.
4. I feel as if I want to go to the toilet all the time.
5. That's OK. It takes a little while to be orientated again after an anaesthetic.
6. Patients who've had abdominal surgery are often in quite a bit of discomfort.
7. I know, but this is very helpful for your recovery quickly.
8. Then I'll put up the head of the bed and let the bed do the work of sitting you up.
9. Remember to take deep breaths and look straight ahead—don't look down, are you ready?
10. And try to move further distance next time; you can use the IV pole to hold onto when you are walking.

Task 1 Pronounce the words.

Write down the words according to the phonetic symbols below. And then listen and check.

1. splenectomy   2. therapy   3. pethidine

4. dextrose   5. analgesia   6. complication

Task 3 Listen and complete.

David Smith, a 36-year-old patient who has had a surgery following a road traffic accident (RTA), comes back to the ward. Mary, the Recovery Nurse, hands David over to Anne, the Ward Nurse. Anne conducts an initial return-to-ward check and starts David on post-op observations. Listen to the conversation and complete the chart below. After that, act it out.
(M=Mary, recovery nurse; A=Anne, ward nurse; D=David, patient.)

M: Hi, Anne. I've got David Smith back from Theatre. Are you taking over his care?

A: Yes, that's me. Hi, David, you're back to the ward now from Recovery. Can you hear me?

D: Mmm.

A: I'll just get a quick handover, and then I'll help make you a bit more comfortable. OK?

M: OK, Anne, I'll just go through the operation report with you. Um, David Smith came in after an RTA. Er, he had the motor bike accident this morning.

A: Ah huh.

M: He's had a splenectomy today at 11: 30 a.m. The operation was uneventful. No post-op complications, except a bit of delayed awakening.

A: Mm. He's still a bit drowsy, isn't he?

M: Yes, a bit. I put him on neuro obs. to notes. His GCS was ten out of fifteen at first. He was opening his eyes to pain, making incomprehensible sounds and obeying commands for movement. When he left Recovery, his GCS was thirteen out of fifteen. He opens his eyes to command. David, can you open your eyes for me?

D: Urgh.

M: That's it. Do you know where you are, David?

D: Um, hospital.

A: That's it. You're back to the ward.

M: Right, his obs. are stable, temp thirty-six, pulse seventy-two, BP one twelve over sixty-four, oxygen sats. are ninety-seven percent on three litres of oxygen.

A: I'll just switch over to our oxygen. David, I'm changing the oxygen tubing over to our wall unit. Can you just breathe normally for me?

D: Mm, yeah. OK.

M: That's it. OK, fluids. He's got a litre of five percent dextrose running.

A: Right. I'll just transfer the bag to our IV stand now. There we are.

M: That litre is due in an hour or so, and there are more fluids written up on the Prescription Chart. Er, David had a few episodes of vomiting post-op, so you might like to keep the IV going for a while. He was given an anti-emetic and he has a prn order in case he had any nausea later on.

A: Great. Er, what about drains?

M: He's got one redivac in situ. David, can I have a look at your drainage tube for a minute?

D: Yeah. OK.

M: Here it is. It's patent. Let's have a look. Yes, it's working well. And it's draining small amounts. It's to be removed when it drains less than twenty millilitres a day.

A: OK.

M: David, can I check the wound now? I'll just take the blanket off for a few minutes. There it is. The wound was closed with clips, as you can see. There are just six clips. The wound's been covered with a non-adhesive dressing (NAD). Leave it intact until reviewed by the surgeon tomorrow, please.

A: OK. Er, what about analgesia?

M: He's been ordered pethidine seventy-five mg IM three hourly for three days, then oral analgesia. He was given pethidine seventy-five mg just before leaving Recovery at, er, 1: 45 p.m. I gave him an extra blanket, too, as he was a bit hypothermic.

A: Right. Thank you. Are you feeling warm enough now, David?

D: Um, yeah. I'm fine. Just sleepy.

A: All right. I'll just put your notes back, and then I'll come and take a few obs. and make you comfortable.

Task 4 Pronounce the words.

Write down the words according to the phonetic symbols below. And then listen and check.

1. hypothermia   2. groggy   3. anaesthetic

4. reaction   5. sensation

Task 5 **Work in pairs.**

Discuss with your partner what will be the appropriate response to patients' complaints. Then listen and check the answer. After that, practise how to respond to the complaints.

A: Morning, David. I'll just do some more obs. and see how you're doing.

D: OK.

A: Temp thirty-six one, pulse sixty-eight, BP a hundred and six over sixty, and your oxygen sats. ninety-six percent on three litres of oxygen. I'll take the oxygen off in a little while, OK? Your temp's still down a bit. Are you warm enough now?

D: *[makes incomprehensible sounds]*

A: So sorry. David. I didn't catch that. I'll just take your mask off for a minute.

D: No, not really. Um, I'm still feeling cold. Is that normal?

A: Yeah, it's OK. It's called hypothermia. It happens sometimes if the operation takes a long time. I'll get you an extra blanket to help warm you up. Are you quite awake after the operation?

D: Yeah, I'm awake now, but I still feel a bit groggy.

A: That's because you've had an anaesthetic. You'll feel better soon.

D: I hope so. My throat feels really sore. It's hard to swallow.

A: Don't worry, that's normal. It's just caused by the tube they put down your throat during the surgery. I'll get you some ice chips to suck soon.

D: Thank you. I don't think I could manage anything else. I feel like I'd be sick if I ate anything.

A: Mm, nausea is sometimes a reaction to post-operative pain. I'll keep an eye on that. How's the pain level now?

D: I'm in bad pain, and everything hurts.

A: That's quite normal. Patients who've had abdominal surgery are often in quite a bit of discomfort. I'll get you an injection for the pain.

D: Good. I feel like I can't move because it's going to be painful.

A: It's quite common to avoid any movement which might cause discomfort, but it's important that I help you to move around and change positions.

D: Oh, I can hardly wait for that! It's strange. I feel as if I want to go to the toilet all the time.

A: It's quite usual to have that sensation, even though you've got a catheter in your bladder. Sometimes the catheter needs a little adjustment so it's more comfortable.

D: I feel dizzy, too. It's like I'm going to fall out of bed.

A: That's OK. It takes a little while to be orientated again after an anaesthetic. I'm going to put these bed rails up while you're feeling a bit wobbly and get you some pain relief. Here's the call bell if you need me.

D: Thank you so much.

Task 7 & **Task 8** **Listen and complete.**

Listen to the conversation and fill in the blanks with the right words.

(N=nurse; J=John, patient)

N: Hello, John. How are you feeling now?

J: Not too great. I feel thirsty.

N: Your doctor told me that you cannot drink anything right now, because you need to give your bowel a rest. Have you passed any gas?

J: No, I don't think so.

N: I can help you gargle, but don't drink it, just rinse and spit it into the emesis basin.

J: By the way, I have a little pain about my incision.

N: Can you stand the pain? If you cannot I will give you some painkillers.

J: Oh. I want to take some painkillers.

N: Now, I'm going to look at your wound and put another dressing on it.

J: OK, be careful.

N: That looks good. In a little while I will be back to get you up.

J: Oh, isn't it too soon to get out of bed?

N: No, as I mentioned before surgery, it is necessary to do it right away so you won't get constipation or lung problems. The first time out of bed I will only get you to the side of the bed. Before we do it, you should move your legs and do some exercises.

(John moves his legs)

N: OK, that's very good. Try again.

J: Oh, my incision hurts.

N: I know, but this is very helpful for your quick recovery.

(A little while later)

N: John, let me help you to get out of bed, maybe you will feel dizzy and light-headed for the first time. Remember to take deep breaths and look straight ahead—don't look down, are you ready?

J: Yes, I guess I am ready.

N: First you need to roll over to your side. Then I'll put up the head of the bed and let the bed do the work of sitting you up. Ok, put your feet over the edge and put your arms on my shoulder. I'll help you sit up. OK, just rest here on the edge. How do you feel?

J: A little woozy.

N: Don't worry. Take some deep breaths. Now I'll help you to stand. Just lift your feet up and down in place here a few times. How do you feel?

J: Just weak.

N: Now we'll walk to the foot of the bed and back.

J: It's not as bad as I expected.

N: Good. Well done. Now back to bed the same way. Sit on the edge of the bed and let yourself down on your side, bring your feet in, and then turn over onto your back.

N: You'd better do it two or three times one day. And try to move further distance next time; you can use the IV pole to hold onto when you are walking.

J: OK, I remember. By the way, when do you think I'll be able to go home?

N: You will be discharged within two weeks; it depends on your progress.

J: That long? What medicine should I take?

N: You should have intravenous antibiotics three times a day. When you can eat and drink you can have the antibiotics orally.

J: Thanks.

N: OK, John. I'll see you later and give you intravenous injection.

Unit 12

Lead-in

Listen and repeat.

Listen to the following sentences and repeat them. Pay attention to the pronunciation and intonation.

1. I'm just going to ask you some questions first so that we can get to know you better. Is that OK?

2. What would you like us to call you?

3. It's your first day here; how do you feel?

4. I understand it's difficult for you at the moment. I hope we can make it easier for you. We're going to try, anyway.

5. Do you have any favourite foods?

6. That's important for us to know, thank you.

7. OK, we'll have to remember that. Anything else you like doing?

8. I see you use a walking stick at home.

9. How about the rest of your mobility? Can you walk to the bathroom by yourself, for example, or do you need to use a commode?

10. You don't wear a hearing aid, so…not hard of hearing. But do you need glasses?

Task 3 Listen and answer.

Listen to a conversation between a nurse and Helen, a new care home resident, and answer the following questions.
(N=nurse; H=Helen, patient)

N: It's Helen, isn't it? When did you arrive?

H: Only a couple of days ago. I'm still getting used to the place. I really miss my own home—my garden and my neighbours, especially.

N: You know, there's a nice little garden here. We could go and sit out there tomorrow if you like.

H: Sounds like a nice idea. Why not?

N: What do you like doing? Do you have any hobbies?

H: I like nature and I read a lot. I saw the TV room yesterday but I don't really like TV any more—I have hearing problems and I don't have the patience to read the subtitles.

N: We organize nature walks, usually in summer. We go for short walks along the beach or into the woods. We also organize day trips to historical sites. And if you like reading, we have a small library with novels and magazines. Why don't you go to the library this afternoon? It's open till 4 p.m.

H: I might do that, thanks. What about Internet access? The manager said there is Internet access.

N: Yes, there is. We have a small computer room. It's a good idea to reserve some time to use the computer. It's more and more popular with the residents. And what about your family? Where do they live?

H: My son and his wife are in Australia, and my daughter lives in Canada. So I keep in contact with them by email. The Internet is very important to me.

N: I can imagine. Listen, it's about time for lunch. Why don't we go into the dining room? I want to introduce you to some of the others.

H: Sure. I was getting hungry.

Task 4 **Listen and check.**

Listen to the first part of a conversation between a nurse and Devin Gyawali, a new care home resident, and choose the correct words in italics in this Assessment Form.

(N=nurse; D=Devin Gyawali, patient)

N: Good afternoon, Mr. Gyawali, nice to meet you. My name's Angela. My team will be taking care of you during your stay at The Beeches.

D: Nice to meet you, too.

N: Now, I'm just going to ask you some questions first so that we can get to know you better. Is that OK?

D: Yes, of course.

N: First question: what would you like us to call you?

D: I prefer people to call me Devin if that's OK.

N: Yes, of course. It's your first day here, Devin. How do you feel?

D: A little sad.

N: Yes? Can you tell me why?

D: I miss my own house, my garden. I like my independence, so you see, I'm…I'm sorry.

N: It's OK. I understand it's difficult for you at the moment. I hope we can make it easier for you. We're going to try, anyway. So, when do you feel happy?

D: That's easy—when I spend time with my family.

N: And who are the children in the photo?

D: My grandchildren, Julie, and that's Peter.

N: Ah, they're beautiful! When did you last see your family?

D: I visited them last month.

N: You can tell me more about them later. What makes you angry?

D: What makes me angry? Well, I don't like people who are impolite or unfriendly.

N: OK. Now, your favourite foods. Do you have any favourite foods?

D: I love Italian and Indian foods, so curry, pasta, that kind of things. And fruits—pineapples, mangoes…

N: Good. Are there any foods you don't like?

D: Bananas—I'm not a fan—and eggs. I am allergic to eggs.

N: That's important for us to know, thank you. Do you wear dentures, by the way?

D: Yes, I do, unfortunately. I hate them.

Task 5 Listen and complete.

Listen to the second part of the conversation and complete the rest of the Assessment Form.

(N=nurse; D=Devin Gyawali, patient)

N: Do you have any hobbies, Devin?

D: Yes, I like sports.

N: Oh, yes. What sports do you follow?

D: I like tennis and cricket—and I usually watch the big games on TV.

N: When will the next big cricket match take place?

D: In the summer.

N: OK, we'll have to remember that. Anything else you like doing?

D: I like music too—classical and traditional Indian music.

N: Do you watch TV, listen to the radio, or read magazines or newspapers?

D: TV for the sports, and I listen to the news on the radio. I don't really read magazines though.

N: I see you use a walking stick at home?

D: Yes, and I used to use a walking frame to go to the shops, for example. I can't walk for a long time without it.

N: OK, that's noted. How about the rest of your mobility? Can you walk to the bathroom by yourself, for example, or do you need to use a commode?

D: No, I don't need a commode but I do find it difficult to pick things up.

N: We can provide you with a grabber if you like. And finally, you don't wear a hearing aid, so…not hard of hearing. But do you need glasses?

D: Yes, I'm short-sighted; I need them for watching TV.

Task 8 Listen and check.

Listen to two elderly people in a care home talking and tick (√) the things that Julie (the first speaker) mentions.

(J=Julie; B=Betty.)

J: …and that nurse—Barbara—I don't like her.

B: Sssh, Julie, she'll hear you!

J: I don't care if she hears me, Betty. She speaks to me like a child—"That's a lovely jumper you're wearing, Julie. Don't you look pretty!" She should call me "Mrs. Taylor", thank you very much! No respect, you see! And she comes into my room without knocking. You've got no privacy, no self-respect.

B: Oh, cheer up. Let's go over and play some bingo.

J: Bingo? I'm not interested in playing bingo with a group of old ladies! It's not very stimulating, is it! They're all so slow because they've got nothing to keep their minds busy, and their medication slows them up some more. They just sit in front of the television all day.

B: Are you coming on the trip to the seaside next week?

J: No, I don't like coach trips. I just want to go home. I miss my independence. I miss my kitchen. And that's another thing—I don't like the food there.

B: Yes, but we don't have to cook or do the washing ourselves. I like this care home. It's clean. The staff are very professional, and it's nice to know there's someone near in an emergency. And there's always someone to talk to. I'm never lonely.

J: Well, I don't want some young nurse telling me what I can and cannot do. I want children around me. It's not natural living like this—everybody here is old!

Unit 13

Lead-in

Listen and repeat.

Listen to the following sentences and repeat them. Pay attention to the pronunciation and intonation.

1. Pregnancy is not a disease, and childbirth is the normal physiological result of completion of pregnancy.

2. Normal delivery can make the mother's womb recover more quickly and better.

3. Cesarean may make the newborn baby hard to breathe.

4. The baby can't be born until the cervix is fully dilated.

5. Open your mouth. Breathe quickly and shallowly.

6. When the next cramp comes, you can start pushing down, just like when you go to the toilet.

7. "Early sucking" means mother-infant skin contact and assists breastfeeding within half an hour after the baby's birth.

8. It is not only economic, simple and with proper temperature, but can also increase the baby's immune function, add the baby's anti-disease capability, and promote the growth of the baby's brain cells.

9. It can also help your uterus recovery, reduce post-partum bleeding, and reduce the chances of breast and ovarian cancer.

10. Let the baby's mouth cover your nipple and most of your areola.

Task 2 Pronounce the words.

Write down the words according to the phonetic symbols below. And then listen and check.

| 1. cesarean | 2. pregnancy | 3. uterus | 4. womb |
| 5. abdomen | 6. dilatation | 7. nauseated | 8. high-risk |

Task 3 Listen and write.

Listen to the sentences and fill in the blanks with the right words.

1. Lying on the left side can increase the blood flow between the uterus and the placenta.

2. The fetus is in a good position and the head is deep engaged.

3. Do you feel the contractions regularly?

4. The cramps are coming more often and are lasting longer.

5. The cervix is open about three centimeters.

6. Your baby will be delivered soon.

Task 4 **Work in pairs.**

Put the following sentences in correct order. Listen and check.

1. My contractions are so close together.

2. Your cervix is fully dilated.

3. It's time to go to the delivery room.

4. Is there a cramp coming?

5. Open your mouth, and breathe quickly and shallowly.

6. When the next cramp comes, you can start pushing down.

7. The head has descended into the vagina.

8. I'm going to make a small surgical incision at the perineum so the delivery will be easier.

Task 5 **Work in pairs.**

Discuss with your partner about how we divide the stages of labour. Then listen and fill in the blanks with the right words.

The first stage—effacement and dilation of cervix: In this stage, and the woman is sociable and excited in latent phase, becoming more inwardly focused on the labour intension.

The second stage—expulsion of fetus: This is a pushing stage, and the woman has intense concentration on pushing, and may doze between contractions.

The third stage—separation of placenta: The woman is excited and relieved after her baby's birth. She is usually very tired.

The fourth stage—physical recovery: 1 to 4 hours after the expulsion of the placenta, the woman is tired, but may find it difficult to rest because of the excitement and eager to be acquainted with the newborn.

Task 6 **Role-play.**

Play the role and listen to the sample.

Sample:

(W=Wang Li, midwife; F=Fang Tong, nurse; M=Mary, patient)

W: Mary, your cervix is fully dilated; it's time to go to the delivery room. Fang Tong, please help her.

F: OK. Mary, you can lean on me. Don't worry!

M: OK, but I feel so dizzy and weak.

W: That's normal. Just sit down on the bed here. Mary, is there a cramp coming? Let's wait until it passes. Open your mouth. Breathe quickly and shallowly. Did the pain go away?

M: I think so.

W: Then you can lie down. Move your buttocks towards the end, and put your feet in the stirrups. When the next cramp comes, you can start pushing down. Wait until you can't hold it any longer and then start pushing down, just like when you go to the toilet.

M: There's another cramp coming.

W: Take a deep breath and push! Push harder! Take another breath and push again! Once more!

F: Oh, I see the baby's crown.

W: Now, I'm going to make a small surgical incision at the perineum so delivery will be easier, and you shouldn't have any serious tears.

F: OK, the head is out! Just one more push and you're done!

W: Congratulations! You have a healthy baby girl! You did a great job!

M: Thank you for your help!

Task 7 **Listen and choose.**

Listen to the dialogue and choose the correct suck posture. And then describe it to your partner.
(M=mother; N=nurse)

M: How should I let the baby suck the milk correctly?

N: You can touch the baby's upper lip with your nipple which will induce the baby's desire for feeding. Let the baby's mouth cover your nipple and most of your areola. Allow the baby to suck the milk slowly and deeply, pause from time to time and swallow the milk with action and sound.

M: How to hold my breast when feeding?

N: Put your fingers together on your chest just below the breast and let your forefinger on the bottom and your thumb on the upper part of your breast. The mother's hand should not be too close to the nipple.

Task 9 **Questions and answers.**

Listen to the dialogue , answer the following questions, and then report to the class.
(M=mother; N=nurse)

M: Oh, the baby is crying. Is she hungry?

N: She is fine, just not familiar with the environment outside. But we can try "early sucking" for her if you feel comfortable.

M: What is "early sucking"?

N: "Early sucking" means mother-infant skin contact and assists breastfeeding within half an hour after birth. It should last no less than 30 minutes. It can stimulate reflection and increase milk secretion.

M: OK, let's try.

N: Let me help you. Look, she is sucking!

M: Yes, she is so cute. But why, I think, I still have no milk?

N: Don't worry, just have the baby suck your nipples and you will be stimulated.

M: Can't I nurse the baby with bottle first?

N: No, it's better to feed a baby with mother's milk. As it's the best natural nutrition for the baby. It is not only economic, simple and with proper temperature, but can also increase the baby's immune function, add the baby's anti-disease capability, and promote the growth of the baby's brain cells. At the same time, it can also help your uterus recovery, reduce post-partum bleeding, and reduce the chances of breast and ovarian cancer. And it can promote the bonding between you and your baby.

M: Oh, there are so many advantages. I will try my best to breastfeed my baby.

N: Good! Your baby is sleeping. Both of you can have a rest, and then you can go back to the ward to see your family soon! The nurse in the ward will provide more breastfeeding guidance for you later.

M: Alright, thanks.

Unit 14

Lead-in

Listen and repeat.

Listen to the following sentences and repeat them. Pay attention to the pronunciation and intonation.

1. You did a good job. / Fabulous. / Good job. / Now you've got it. / You tried hard. / You are on top of it. / Super job.

2. You're improving. / You are on target. / You're on your way. / You're making progress.

3. Don't rush. / No rush. There's plenty of time.

4. Tell me if it hurts.

5. Your body needs the nutrition so that you can regain your strength and energy.

6. I have noticed that you have fought to recover in such a determined way.

7. It's common after the shock of such a big car accident.

8. Long stay in bed may make you lose confidence.

9. You have done very well considering the extent of your injuries.

10. I think we could stop here.

Task 2 Pronounce the words.

Write down the words according to the phonetic symbols below. And then listen and check.

1. occupational	2. therapy	3. treatment	4. physiotherapy
5. joint	6. muscle	7. nerve	8. massage

Task 3 Listen and check.

Listen to the audio and complete the steps of guiding a patient in recovery exercises.

Guiding a patient in recovery exercises. First explain the benefits and procedure of the exercise. Then set the goals according to the patient's health status. Last but not least, encourage the patient.

Task 5 Work in pairs.

Listen to a nurse helping Anita, a patient who is recovering from a stroke, with meal. Pay attention to the nurse's expressions of encouragement and comforting words used in the conversation, and put a tick (√) in the column. Then repeat it.

(N=nurse; P=patient)

N: Hello Anita, here is your lunch.

P: I don't feel like eating.

N: Do you feel sick or any discomfort?

P: No…I don't feel sick, but I hate to sit here for the whole day. It seems I can't do anything after the stroke. I can even hardly feed myself… I just don't have appetite at all.

N: I can really understand that you don't feel hungry. But your body needs the nutrition so that you can regain your strength and energy. I've got some tools to help you. Maybe you can try and eat on your own.

P: OK…I will try and eat a little bit.

N: These are non-slip bowl and no spill cup.

P: Em… They are good.

N: There are some modified utensils for you, too.

P: What for?

N: These spoons are easier for you to hold.

P: Right, well. I'll try them out.

(Patient eats some of her meal.)

N: You did really well. Did you finish your meal? Or you would like to have some other food?

P: I have done with the meal.

N: May I take these utensils away?

(Patient nods.)

N: I could see that was hard work for you, but you did a good job. You have eaten half of the meal on your own!

P: Thank you.

Task 8 Listen and complete.

Listen and tick "√" the ROM exercises the patient can do in 1-6, and circle the correct words in 7-10.

(N=nurse; P=patient)

N: Hi Theresa, it's important to do these exercises every day. Our goal is two sets of eight on shoulders and elbows.

P: All right. I'll try. I think my right shoulder is getting stronger. I can lift my right arm during dinner.

N: That's good to hear. Let's try the right shoulder first. Ready?

P: OK, yes.

N: Please lift your right upper arm up as far as you can. That's right. You are doing quite well. Now move back. And repeat that. Good, very good. One more…again…relax. Very good. Now let's try to move your right shoulder in a rotated motion…repeat four times in each direction…a little higher… fabulous! A little rest?

P: I'm fine. Thank you.

N: Now extend your right elbow as far as you can. Tell me if it hurts.

P: OK…

N: …then back.

P: Ouch!

N: Do you feel pain?

P: I'm fine. I can stand it.

N: Don't push yourself too hard. Relax and slow down. Still want to try?

P: Yes.

N: Let's count together. One, two, three... You are doing really well! Now for the left shoulder. Are you ready?

P: Yes.

N: Please lift you left upper arm up as far as you can...

P: That's my limit.

N: OK...120 degrees. Do you want the shoulder extension exercise?

P: I'm so sorry. I feel tired.

N: I think we'd better stop now. It's much better than yesterday.

P: Yes, Thank you.

Unit 15

Lead-in

Listen and repeat.

Listen to the following sentences and repeat them. Pay attention to the pronunciation and intonation.

1. Dr. Sim informed us that you were going home today, so I will remove your IV catheter and make a discharge plan for you.

2. It's a good idea to install grab bars around the bath, so she can hold them as she gets in and out of the bath.

3. If you get a raised toilet seat, you'll be able to slide from your wheelchair onto the toilet.

4. Lidia's daughter asked if you could let her know what time the home assessment's being done so she can come over to her mother's house.

5. The doctor has prescribed some medications for you; I just want to talk to you about them.

6. First, avoid any mental stress and have a good rest.

7. Secondly, examinations of fasting blood sugar and an ECG should be done regularly.

8. You need to keep the dressing on until you have your sutures removed.

9. I'm afraid I can't talk to you about your father's results because of confidentiality.

10. If you feel that there are any complications/problems, please contact the hospital immediately.

Task 2 Listen and complete.

The discharged patient's current ADLs (Activities of Daily Living) Assessment is a part of the Discharge Plan. Listen to a dialogue about a nurse going through a patient's Discharge Plan for the independence assessment. Tick (√) the correct boxes in the following assessment form.

(N=nurse; A=Amy, patient)

N: So, Amy, we're going to look at your Discharge Plan together. I'm going to explain what's going to happen and if you have any questions, just ask, OK?

A: Nurse, I live alone and I am not sure if I'll manage myself at home.

N: Do you have a friend or family member who can help you?

A: I know my sister will help me if I have problems and maybe my neighbour, if necessary.

N: That's good. How do you feel about getting to the toilet and getting dressed by yourself?

A: I think I'll be OK, I've been managing by myself with the toilet and I can get dressed if things are easy to reach.

N: Can your sister prepare your clothes for you every evening?

A: Yes, I suppose she can. What about washing? I'm worried I'll fall if I'm not careful.

N: Be sure to put a non-slip mat in the shower and maybe a couple of grab bars as well.

A: Grab bars? What are they?

N: You put them around the shower and you can hold on to them to stop yourself from slipping.

A: Oh, OK, I see. That's a good idea.

N: How about preparing meals? Are you worried about that?

A: Yes, that's the thing I'm most worried about. If I feel as tired as I am today, I won't have the energy for cooking.

N: That's true. If you start feeling tired, make sure you rest, that's very important. Try to eat at least one piece of fruit every day and drink lots of water. But perhaps your sister can prepare some meals in advance? You can heat them up when you want.

A: Uh huh.

N: Now, you can't drive again for another three to four weeks. If you need help with the shopping, will your neighbour do it, perhaps?

A: Yes, I'm sure he will.

Task 4 Work in pairs.

Put these words in order to make sentences. Discuss what the instructions are about by writing the number in the box below. Then listen and check.

1. The staff nurse has already sent your prescription to the pharmacy.

2. Let me check about your follow-up appointment with the doctor.

3. Have regular meals and keep a diet of vegetables and fruits.

4. Which exercise should I take?

5. Your follow-up appointment has been made for 10 a.m. Wednesday.

6. Continue your low-salt diet after your discharge.

7. Take a tablespoonful three times a day at mealtimes.

8. What are aerobic exercise?

Task 5 Work in pairs.

The nurse is having conversations with three of her patients on their discharge. Listen to the three dialogues. What are the patients/caregivers worried about? Tick (√) the correct answer in the box below. What mobility aid(s) does the nurse recommend? Write down the answer in the right column. Then students work in pairs to have conversations about giving advice on mobility aids. Use the sentence patterns below to help you.

1.

(N=nurse; B=Mr. Black, patient)

N: Your wife is very frail, Mr. Black. And she's going to need help with going to the toilet, for example.

B: Yes, I realize that. But it's going to be difficult for me to lift her on and off the toilet.

N: Yes. If you get a raised toilet seat, she'll be able to slide from her wheelchair onto the toilet. That'll make it easier for you, too.

B: Erm, that's a good idea, I'll look into it.

2.

(N=nurse; M=Mary, patient)

N: Your mother will need help getting in and out of the bath.

M: Yes, I'm a bit worried about that. She'll fall if she's not careful; I know what she's like.

N: It's a good idea to install grab bars around the bath, so she can hold on to them as she gets in and out of the bath. And if she has a non-slip mat, it'll stop her from slipping. Does she have one?

M: No.

N: I strongly advise you to get one. They're not expensive.

M: You're right. If we have time, we'll visit the local DIY store on the way home and get one.

3.

(N=nurse; J=Jim, patient)

N: So, Jim, you're leaving tomorrow. Good news!

J: I know. It's too cool!

N: So how do you feel about washing and dressing? Do you feel strong enough to do this by yourself today? You need to practise before we discharge you.

J: Yeah, sure, why not? I'll give it a go. But if I stand for a long time, I get tired.

N: Well, there's a shower chair in the bathroom. Why don't you take your shower after sitting down today? If you need help, just press the buzzer.

Task 6 Role-play.

Listen to the sample. Play the roles of the sample or play the roles following the role card below.

(N=nurse; S=Susan, patient)

N: Good Morning, Susan. How are you feeling today?

S: Fine, thanks. I feel great today.

N: Congratulations! Here is a discharge form for you.

S: That's good news! You see I'm really looking forward to going back to work.

N: Don't be in a hurry.

S: How long do you think it will be before I can return to my work?

N: I can assure you that you'll fully recover in three to five weeks.

S: Is there anything I should follow?

N: You'd better have a good rest for one week.

S: You mean I should stay in bed for the whole week?

N: You should go outdoors more and do some exercise.

S: What kind of food should I have, special nourishment?

N: Have regular meals first. Keep a diet of vegetables and fruits. Keep off alcohol. If possible, give up smoking, at least for a time.

S: Should I take some medicines?

N: Yes, your doctor has written a prescription for you. You have to take them every day.

S: When will these tablets be finished?

N: In a week.

S: How should they be taken?

N: Take one tablet of this medicine three times a day before meals. And that one, two tablets once daily in the morning.

S: I see. Thank you.

N: Remember to come to the Out-patient Department for a consultation; your follow-up appointment with Dr. Milton is in a week.

S: All right.

N: You can pack your things and settle the account today.

S: All right, but I must inform my husband first.

N: I have called him for you. He is coming in half an hour.

S: I feel really grateful to you. Many thanks.

N: You are welcome. We wish you an early recovery. Goodbye.

Task 8 & Task 9 Listen and complete.

Sandy, the Ward Nurse, makes a telephone referral to the District Nursing Service on a patient's discharge. Listen to the conversation and complete the sections marked 1-10.

(M=Milly, District Nurse; S=Sandy, hospital registered nurse)

M: District Nursing Service. Milly Frank speaking.

S: Hello, it's Sandy here from the Alexandra Hospital. I've got an 80-year-old lady I'd like to refer to you for some District Nursing Services. Can I give you the details now?

M: Could you hold on for a minute? I'll get a referral form. OK, I'm ready, er, it was Sandy, wasn't it?

S: That's right. Sandy Clarke from the Alexandra Hospital.

M: Thanks, Sandy. What's the patient's name, please?

S: I've got a Linda Gilbert for you.

M: OK. Could you please spell that for me?

S: Sure. It's L-I-N-D-A, the surname's spelled G-I-L-B-E-R-T.

M: Got it. Linda Gilbert.

S: Her address is 15 Summer Lane, Exeter. It's a bungalow. The spare key's with her next of kin.

M: OK, do you have Linda's home phone number, please?

S: Yes, I've got it here. It's o one two five four, five five six, seven two three.

M: Yes, thanks. O one two five four, five five six, seven two three. Is that correct?

S: Yes, that's right. Do you want me to give you her daughter's number, too?

M: Yes, please.

S: Her daughter's name is Andrea. She is also her next of kin. Her phone number is o one four five six, six seven nine, nine nine eight.

M: Got it. Thanks.

S: Linda's GP is Dr. John Hockings. I'll spell that for you. It's H-O-C-K-I-N-G-S.

M: OK.

S: Linda had a stroke three weeks ago. She's got moderate left-sided weakness and still has some difficulty in swallowing. She needs quite a lot of help with her ADLs, especially bathing and mobility. She's quite unsteady on her feet and uses a walking frame.

M: What will I have to order?

S: She might need a shower chair. But it'd be better to wait until after she has a home assessment done before any aids are ordered. The home assessment has been booked for 12th June.

M: That's Monday, 12th June, right?

S: Yes, that's it. Linda's house will need some adaptions.

M: OK. How's she managed with her diet?

S: She's been managing a soft diet for a few days.

M: Mm, soft diet. Does she need her meals delivered to her at home?

S: No. Her daughters are very supportive. Well, I think I've given you all the information you need. Her discharge summary will be sent to you in the next day or so. Is there anything else you need to know?

M: No. I think I've got everything. Thanks.

S: No problem and thanks for your help.

教学基本要求

一、课程性质和课程任务

《护理英语（听说分册）》主要面向高职高专护理、助产及医学相关专业。根据《高等职业学校护理专业教学标准》和《高职高专教育英语课程教学基本要求（试行）》"以实用为主，以应用为目的"的要求，本教材旨在结合岗位的需求分析，提高学生的医护专业英语口语能力，特别是学生同病患、病患家属或其他医务工作者沟通的行业英语的口语表达能力，让学生胜任国内普通医院、外资医疗机构的涉外医护工作，甚至能在国际医护专业市场找到一席之地。

本教材可供护理、助产及医学相关专业使用，希望能在教学中体现可操作性。本教材围绕章节主题，设计多个任务，以听力任务为辅，为学生做好语言输入和积累；以口语任务为主，完成工作场景中可能遇到的模拟任务（如采集病史、生命体征测量、交班、用药指导等）。

二、课程教学目标

课程目标分三大类：知识、技能和素养目标，努力实现三位一体，相互支撑。

◇ 知识目标：以实用为主制定教学目标，即学生通过这门课的学习能够用英语描绘（包括书面和口头）常见的医护情景，熟悉各种医护专业术语的英语表达方式。

◇ 技能目标：学会使用英语采集病史，交班，交流等。初步学会医护专业学生应具备的医护英语知识和医护英语听说技能。

◇ 素养目标：培养学生热爱专业，具有人文关怀的精神、高度的工作责任心和高尚的职业道德；培养把专业知识融入英语学习的能力；培养具有扎实的英语语言基础知识和技能、丰富的医护专业英语和临床专业知识与技能，能够在合资/外资医疗机构、国外医疗机构等从事涉外医护工作的复合型人才。

三、学时分配建议（60 学时）

建议护理专业的学生学习所有的章节，其他专业的学生可根据实际情况选择相关内容学习。

序号（章节）	教学内容	学时数		
		理论	实践	合计
1	Admitting Patients	1	3	4
2	Taking Vital Signs	1	3	4
3	Researching Symptoms	1	3	4
4	Collecting Samples	1	3	4
5	Talking about Pain	1	3	4
6	Administering Medicine	1	3	4
7	Giving IV	1	3	4
8	Performing Hygienic Care	1	3	4

序号（章节）	教学内容	学时数		
		理论	实践	合计
9	Talking about Nutrition	1	3	4
10	Caring for Pre-operative Patients	1	3	4
11	Caring for Post-operative Patients	1	3	4
12	Caring for the Elderly	1	3	4
13	Caring for Obstetric Patients	1	3	4
14	Helping Patients with Rehabilitation	1	3	4
15	Discharging Patients	1	2	3

Suggested Answers

Unit 1

Communication Focus

1. The work of a receptionist in hospital is to greet and assist patients when they arrive, make appointments for patients, record patients' information, and file patients' records. Hospital receptionists have to operate the computer, a fax machine and other office equipment. Besides, they also have to know about first aid, and understand medical technology and abbreviations.

2. Good morning, my name is Cindy, the nurse in charge of this department. I'll admit you to the ward. How do you prefer to be addressed? …Now, I'd like to collect your personal information, is that OK with you? …

Part One

Task 1

1. g	2. f	3. h	4. d
5. e	6. a	7. b	8. c

Descriptions:

1. In the Nurse Station, nurses and other healthcare staff work behind the counter when not working directly with patients and they can perform some of their duties.

2. In the Operating Room, patients will be given operations.

3. In the Consulting Room, a patient will be asked questions about his/her problems which bring him/her to the hospital.

4. Pharmacy is a department in hospital of preparing and dispensing drugs.

5. Medical Department focuses on the programmes involving internal medicine, including cancer, heart disease, kidney disease, diabetes, endocrine disorder, pulmonary problem and geriatric problem.

6. A Ward is a department or room of a hospital set aside for a particular class or group of patients.

7. Surgical Department is a medical specialty that uses operative manual and instrumental techniques on a patient to investigate or treat a pathological condition such as a disease or injury, to help in improving bodily function or appearance or to repair unwanted ruptured areas.

8. Emergency Room in a hospital is staffed and equipped to provide emergency care to persons requiring immediate medical treatment.

Task 2

1. emergency	2. pediatrics	3. surgery
4. maternity	5. geriatrics	6. radiology

Task 3

1. children   2. operations   3. emergency cases
4. take X-rays   5. babies   6. elderly

Part Two

Task 4

3   8   5   9   4   1   6   2   7

Task 5

1. Good morning, Caroline. I'm sorry to trouble you so much.

2. Welcome, Mrs. Johnson. I'm Daisy, the nurse in charge of this department.

3. Would you mind if I check out some details of you?

4. What would you like to know?

5. I'd like to check your name and date of birth.

6. My full name is Catherine Jonathan and the date of my birth is the fifth of July, nineteen fifty-seven.

7. I'll bring you to your bedside. Please follow me.

8. We supply hot water and the toilet is over there.

9. Please let us know if you need any help.

10. Smoking is not allowed here.

Task 6

Sample:

(N=nurse; P=patient)

N: Good morning Madam, I'd like to check your personal details, is that okay?

P: Yes, of course.

N: Could you tell me your full name, please?

P: Catherine Miller.

N: Can you spell that, please?

P: C-A-T-H-E-R-I-N-E, Catherine, M-I-L-L-E-R, Miller.

N: All right, and what would you like us to call you?

P: Catherine is fine.

N: Well, Catherine, where are you from?

P: I'm originally from Chicago. But I came here for my studies. I got married, and now I'm looking forward to my first child. I've been here for ten years already.

N: That's lovely, and what is your date of birth?

P: The 20th of August,1982.

N: Is that the 20th of August,1982?

P: That's right.

N: And what is your job?

P: Advertising manager for Bxx company.

N: Advertising manager. Okay, I also need to ask who your next of kin is to contact in an emergency.

P: My husband, Daniel Miller, is my next of kin. His mobile number is 0677-998-7787.

N: Thank you. Do you have any allergies?

P: No.

Part Three

Task 7

A

1.The name of the patient is Richard Stewart.

2. The patient is a man.

3. It's the twenty-first of February, nineteen eighty-two.

4. He's a supermarket manager.

5.Dr. Phillip is Richard's family doctor.

B

1. GP

2. DOB

3. allergies

4. M/F

5. occupation

6. marital status

7. medical history

8. next of kin

9. n/a

Task 8

ID Bracelet	
Full name	Allen Cooper
DOB	20/08/1947
Hospital NO.	767837
Allergy	Penicillin
Next of kin	Daughter, Katherine Cooper
Contact NO.	94770077579

Task 9

A

Patient Detail	
Name	Marilyn Stuart
Gender	Female

DOB	12/7/1979
Country of origin	America
Job	Fashion designer
Next of kin	Edison Stuart
Relationship with the patient	Husband
Allergy	Morphine

B

Sample:

(E=Emma, nurse; M=Marilyn Stuart, patient)

E: Welcome Mrs. Stuart. I'm the nurse in charge of this department. My name is Emma. I need to get some information from you. Would you mind if I ask you some questions?

M: No, that's fine.

E: Thank you. First I need to know your full name.

M: My name is Marilyn Stuart.

E: And can you tell me your date of birth?

M: Yes, the twelfth of July, nineteen seventy-nine.

E: Well, where do you come from?

M: I'm an American. I came here for my studies seven years ago. And now I'm a fashion designer in a boutique.

E: That's lovely. I'd like to know who your next of kin is.

M: I'm married, and my husband, Edison Stuart is my next of kin.

E: Okay, one more question. Do you have any allergies?

M: Oh, yes. I'm allergic to morphine.

E: Thank you, Mrs. Stuart. That's all for me.

M: Thanks, Emma.

More Practice

Sample:

(N=nurse; G=Mr. Green, patient)

N: Good morning, Mr. Green. I'm the nurse in charge of this department. I'll get some information about you. What's your full name, please?

G: My full name is Jim Green.

N: Could you tell me the date of your birth and job?

G: Sure. It's 17th July 1959. And I'm a taxi driver.

N: What brings you here today?

G: Well, I've got a terrible cough and I'm experiencing pain when I cough.

N: How long has all this been going on?

G: Um…about half a month.

N: Do you have a history of chest infection?

G: Yes, I was admitted to hospital with bronchitis last year.

N: Oh, are you a smoker?

G: Yes, I am. Actually, I'm a heavy smoker. I usually have 3 packs of cigarettes a day. I have smoked for 30 years and often have a chest infection.

N: I see. Could I collect some information about your family?

G: Sure. Go ahead.

N: Well. Where do you live and who do you live with?

G: I live on 27 May Avenue, Santa David Street. My wife who is 52 years old and my three teenage children live with me.

N: Do you have any other health problems?

G: No, I have no other problems bothering me.

N: Have you ever tried giving up smoking?

G: Yes, I've tried stopping smoking several times, but I failed.

N: Have you attended any smoking-quit program?

G: No, I haven't. Do you have any good suggestions?

N: Firstly, reduce smoking times per day gradually. Secondly, take regular exercises. Thirdly, do not work too hard and have more water or juice.

G: Thank you for your suggestions.

N: You're welcome. You can have a rest now. Let me know if you need any help.

Unit 2

Communication Focus

1. Because obtaining a patient's consent before performing healthcare procedures is not just a matter of common courtesy, but indeed a legal healthcare requirement in Western native English-speaking countries.

2. Use verbal language, like "I'm going to…, is that alright with you?"

Part One

Task 1

1. kg	2. %	3. RR	4. P
5. T	6. O_2Sats	7. BP	8. Wt.

Task 2

1. heart rate	2. pulse	3. blood pressure	4. respiratory
5. temperature	6. oxygen	7. saturation	8. observation

Task 3

1. BP	2. T	3. P	4. RR	5. T

Part Two

Task 4

1. d   2. b   3. i   4. f   5. c

6. g   7. h   8. e   9. a

1. A stethoscope is used by a nurse to listen to heart sounds.

2. A tympanic thermometer is used to measure a patient's ear/tympanic membrane temperature.

3. A BP cuff is wrapped around the patient's upper arm when we take his blood pressure.

4. A mercury sphygmomanometer is used to measure a patient's blood pressure.

5. A pulseoximeter is used to measure how much oxygen there is in a patient's blood—the oxygen saturation. And it can also be used to take pulse.

6. An electronic thermometer is used to measure a patient's, esp. a child's body temperature.

7. A watch with second hand is used when we count a patient's pulse and respiratory rate.

8. A glass mercury thermometer is used to take a patient's body temperature, esp. oral and rectal temperature.

9. A digital blood pressure monitor is used to measure a patient's blood pressure.

Task 5

1. Can you hold your arm out straight for me? (blood pressure)

2. Just pop this under your tongue. (temperature)

3. I'll put this probe into your ear. (temperature)

4. Can I have your wrist, please? (pulse)

5. Can you roll up your sleeve? (blood pressure)

6. Please put your finger into this probe. (oxygen saturation & pulse)

7. Just breathe in and out normally. (respiratory rate)

8. Can you give me your right hand, please? (pulse)

Task 6

Sample:

(N=nurse; P=patient)

N: Ms. Smith, I'm going to take your obs. now. Is that OK?

P: Sure, go ahead.

N: Did you drink any hot water in the last half an hour?

P: No, I didn't.

N: OK, let me take your temperature first. Please put this thermometer under your armpit for a short while; and keep your arm firmly up against your chest until I take it out.

P: (*Takes the thermometer and puts it under the armpit.*) Is that right?

N: Yes, good. Have you been smoking, drinking coffee or taking any kind of stimulants today?

P: No, I haven't.

N: Well, I'm just going to take your pulse; can I have your wrist, please?

P: (*Stretches the arm on the table.*)

N: (*Looks at the watch and counts the pulse and respiration. And after finishing measuring them, writes down the readings.*)

P: How is my pulse?

N: Your pulse is sixty-five beats per minute. And I've also checked your respiration. It is eighteen breaths per minute.

P: Are they normal?

N: Yes, they are quite normal. Now, please give me the thermometer.

P: Here you are. Do I have a temperature?

N: (*Writes down the number on the chart.*) It is thirty-eight point three degrees Celsius, a little high. Before I take your blood pressure, could you please tell me if you have had any previous surgery done on either your chest or arms?

P: No.

N: Do you have any history of high blood pressure?

P: No, never.

N: Ok. Ms. Smith, please roll up the sleeve of your left arm, and lift your arm a little so I can put on the blood pressure cuff.

P: (*Rolls up the sleeve and lifts the arm on the table.*)

N: (*Wraps the cuff around the arm and then inflates the cuff.*) When I inflate the blood pressure cuff, it'll be a little tight. (*Notes down the measurement on the chart.*) Your blood pressure is good, one hundred over eighty; it's in the normal range.

P: That's good.

N: All right. That's all for me. I'll report all the results to the doctor.

P: Thank you, nurse.

N: You are welcome.

Part Three

Task 7

1. d	2. f	3. b	4. c	5. e	6. a

Task 8

Observation Chart				U / N: 201984 Surname: Carter Given names: Felton DOB: 22/9/1945 Sex: Male			
Date	**Time**	**T**	**P**	**R**	**BP**	**Comment**	**Signature**
2/3/2017	02:00	1. 36.5	2. 86	18	3. 175/102		J. Perez
2/3/2017	06:00	36.4	4. 76	16	5. 176/95		J. Perez
2/3/2017	10:00	36.4	6. 112	7. 22	8. 210/130		J. Perez
2/3/2017	14:00	36.3	9. 97	20	10. 185/90		J. Perez
2/3/2017	15:00	36.5	11. 86	18	12. 170/85		J. Perez

Observation Chart					U / N: 201975 Surname: Castle Given names: Rosa DOB: 9/2/1968 Sex: Female		
Date	**Time**	**T**	**P**	**R**	**BP**	**Comment**	**Signature**
2/3/2017	06:00	37.3	72	13.18	130/90		J. Perez
2/3/2017	07:00	37.5	76	18	105/65		J. Perez
2/3/2017	08:00					OT	J. Perez
2/3/2017	09:00					OT	J. Perez
2/3/2017	10:00					OT	J. Perez
2/3/2017	11:00					OT	J. Perez
2/3/2017	12:00					OT	J. Perez
2/3/2017	13:00					OT	J. Perez
2/3/2017	14:00	37.2	78	14.26	120/75		J. Perez
2/3/2017	15:00	37.4	76	15.20	115/65		J. Perez

Task 9

Sample:

All right, now I'll just let you know about Gladys Small's vital signs. Mrs. Small was admitted before 7:00 a.m. today with poorly managed hypertension and low fever. On admission, her temperature was thirty-eight nine degrees Celsius and her BP was one seventy over one ten at 7:00 a.m. Both of them were higher than normal. Her pulse was one hundred and respiration was eighteen. Both of them were normal. At 12:35, her temperature went down to thirty seven nine degrees Celsius, but she still had a slight fever. Her pulse decreased to ninety. It was still in normal range. Her BP also went up to two hundred over one twenty. It was very high. Then she was given IV as ordered. Her respiration remained the same.

At 3:00 p.m., her temperature fell to thirty-seven two degrees Celsius and pulse decreased to eighty-six. Both of them were normal. Her respiration stabilised. Her BP went down to one forty over ninety. It was finally normal, but it still needs to be aware of.

More Practice

Sample:

(S=Susan, nures; F=Mr. Ford, patient)

S: Hello, Mr. Ford. I'm Susan.

F: Hello, Susan.

S: What brought you here to the A&E unit?

F: I got a terrible injury over my knee.

S: Oh, I'm sorry. But what happened?

F: You know, I'm a physical trainer at the gym. This morning when I was doing a somersault, I slipped and fell down off the ground, and my right knee was severely injured.

S: I see. Now I'm going to take your vital signs. Is that OK with you?

F: It's OK.

(After taking Mr. Ford's vital signs.)

F: Are my vital signs normal?

S: Your temperature and respirations are fine. But your pulse rate seems to be below the average rate for an adult. Your pulse is 48 beats per minute. And the normal range for a healthy adult is between 60 and 100.

F: Is it serious?

S: Don't worry too much. You are a physical trainer, aren't you?

F: Yes, so what?

S: Professional athlete often has a slower pulse rate than the average person does, even at rest. So there is a strong probability that your slow pulse rate is quite normal for you. Do you have any other complaints apart from your painful knee?

F: No, I feel fine.

S: Do you know what your pulse rate normally is?

F: Actually I can't remember my previous readings, but nothing showed abnormal in my regular check-ups.

S: OK. I will write down your reading on the Obs. Chart. To make sure that you don't have anything wrong with your pulse, I'm coming to take your pulse every two hours.

F: Hope there isn't anything wrong.

S: Don't worry. I will inform the nurse in charge of your condition. We are going to take good care of you.

F: Thank you, Susan.

S: You're welcome. Just feel at home here.

Unit 3

Communication Focus

1. RN: At present you have a clot which is blocking one of your heart arteries and causing this heart attack. We are going to give you a drug now that should break the clot down and improve the blood flow to your heart muscle.

2. RN: We are just going to start you on a heparin infusion now. It is a continuous drip we give you which will thin your blood and prevent further clots from occurring.

Part One

Task 1

| a. 9 | b. 8 | c.10 | d. 5 | e. 3 |
| f. 1 | g. 2 | h. 4 | i. 6 | j. 7 |

1. I think fever is among the top five because when we get some infections our body temperature will rise. And infections are common and sometimes serious.

2. I think sore throat is among the top five, because it often occurs in the cold season of a year. Viral infection is the main cause for that.

3. I think stomachache is among the top five, because the acute stomachache affects one's normal life.

4. I think breathlessness is among the top five, because breathlessness will put you at risk for a death.

5. I think rashes are among the top five, because skin rashes will spread to the eye and the skin irritation, or even causing respiratory problems.

Task 2

1. b   2. a   3. c   4. e   5. d

Task 3

1. N: How long have you had the pain in your belly?

2. N: Has it moved again?

3. N: Does the characteristic of the pain change?

4. N: Have you had any diarrhea?

5. N: Did you have a fever?

Part Two

Task 4

1. He has a severe headache.

2. He is suffering from an acute bad headache.

3. Maybe he has to buy some pain killers first and has an EEG test and an MRI scan.

Task 5

1. head	2. bad headache	3. left part	4. sickness
5. vision	6. flashing lights	7. eyes	8. dizzy
9. hearing	10. numbness		

Task 6

Sample:

(M=mother; N=nurse; C=child)

M: My child has a temperature, a headache, a sore throat and a rash.

N: How long has he been ill?

M: He's had the temperature since yesterday.

N: Are there any sick children in the neighborhood or at school?

M: One of his classmates had a fever and complained of a sore throat five days ago.

N: *(Turns to the child)* Let me have a look. Open your mouth and show me your tongue. Say Ah……

C: Ah.

N: *(Uses the tongue depressor and penlight to check the child's mouth.)* Now take off your clothes.

M: What have you found?

N: His tonsils are swollen and red. His tongue is as red as a strawberry. There is a rash all over his body.

N: He may need a blood test. Go to the Pathology Department for it and bring the result here, please.

(Thirty minutes later.)

M: Here is the result. Is it normal?

N: His white blood cell count is high. He is probably suffering from scarlet fever.

M: What kind of disease is it?

N: It is a kind of infectious disease. You should keep him away from other children as much as possible.

M: What can I do for him?

N: He should stay in bed until his fever goes down. Let him eat easily digestible food and drink plenty of fluid.

M: Does he need to take some drugs?

N: I'll tell the doctor and he will prescribe penicillin injections for a few days.

M: What should I do about his rash?

N: You should prevent him from scratching it.

M: OK. Thank you.

Part Three

Task 7

Last night Miss Miller had a car accident and bled a lot. She had lost consciousness for a while. Later she was admitted **to the** hospital and was given an injection of 5ml tetanus toxoid by the nurse. Today she is not feeling any pain. She is supposed to **be** (删除) support **ed** (删除) the cast and body with pillows in good alignment and keep the cast uncover **ed.** Any sign of decreased circulation, coldness, swelling or numbness should be reported.

Task 8

Yesterday Mr. Williams had a mild fever and complained of a loss of appetite. Later he suffered from nausea and vomiting with an occasional pain in the center of his stomach. He was admitted to the hospital yesterday with severe abdominal pain. This morning his abdomen is swollen and he is suffering from a constant sharp pain in his lower right side of his abdomen.

Task 9

Sample:

AIDS:

Acquired immune deficiency syndrome (AIDS) is a spectrum of conditions caused by infection with the human immunodeficiency virus (HIV). Following initial infection, a person may not notice any symptoms or may experience a brief period of influenza-like illness.

About 40% to 90% of people have flu-like symptoms within 2-4 weeks after HIV infection. Other people do not feel sick at all during the early stage, which is also known as acute HIV infection. Early infection is defined as HIV infection in the past six months (recent) and includes acute (very recent) infections. Flu-like symptoms can include: fever, chills, rash, night sweats, muscle aches, sore throat, fatigue, swollen lymph nodes, mouth ulcers and etc.

Tuberculosis:

Tuberculosis (TB) is an infectious disease usually caused by the bacterium Mycobacterium tuberculosis (MTB). Tuberculosis generally affects the lungs, but can also affect other parts of the body. Most infections do not have symptoms, in which case it is known as latent tuberculosis. About 10% of latent infections progress to active disease which, if left untreated, kills about half of those infected. The classic symptoms of active TB are a chronic cough with blood-containing sputum, fever, night sweats, and weight loss. The historical term "consumption" came about due to the weight loss. Infection of other organs can cause a wide range of symptoms.

Leprosy:

Leprosy, also known as Hansen's disease (HD), is a long-term infection by the bacterium Mycobacteriumleprae or Mycobacteriumlepromatosis. Initially, infections are without symptoms and typically remain this way for 5 to 20 years. Symptoms that develop include granulomas of the nerves, respiratory tract, skin, and eyes. This may result in a lack of ability to feel pain, thus loss of parts of extremities due to repeated injuries or infection due to unnoticed wounds. Weakness and poor eyesight may also be present.

More Practice

Sample:

N: How were you injured?

P: I have had a car accident, banging my forehead quite hard. My wife wrapped a bandage around it to stop the bleeding.

N: Did you lose a lot of blood?

P: Not too much.

N: Were you unconscious?

P: For about a couple of minutes, I think, I lost consciousness.

N: The wound is rather large, so I will stitch it up.

P: Will it hurt?

N: Oh, no. It won't be painful. We'll give you a local anesthetic. You're a brave fellow. Well, we're all finished.

N: Have you had an anti-tetanus injection lately?

P: I think the only one I had was about 5 years ago.

N: Well, I think you'd better have another one.

P: Whatever you say.

(After the shot.)

N: Ok, it's done. Since you have hurt your head, I'm afraid you must stay in hospital tonight for further observation. If you feel anything wrong, just tell me.

P: All right.

Unit 4

Communication Focus

1. Because it is not only an effective way of minimizing patients' anxiety, but also more likely to enhance their compliance with the instruction.

2. Firstly, the nurse should understand what the patient actually knows about the healthcare that he is going to undertake.

   Secondly, the nurse gives explanations and education in patients' languages.

   Thirdly, the nurse clarifies whether the patients understand or not by their feedback.

Part One

Task 1

1. Urine Test　　　　　　2. Stool (Feces) Test　　　　　　3. Blood Test

Task 2

Urine　　d. e		a. a problem in the intestine	
		b. diabetes	
Blood　　b. c		c. liver inflammation	
		d. infection in the bladder	
Stool (Feces)　　a		e. infection in the kidneys	

Task 3

1. urine	2. diabetes	3. stool	4. feces
5. intestine	6. infection	7. bladder	8. kidney

Part Two

Task 4

2	a. cotton stick	1	b. tourniquet	3	c. needle	4	d. specimen tube

1. Tourniquet is a band of cloth or rubber that is twisted tightly around an injured arm or leg to stop bleeding.

2. Cotton stick is capable of storing liquid medicine (disinfectant or therapeutic liquid medicine) with controllable medicine dose.

3. Needle is a very thin, pointed steel tube at the end of a syringe, which is pushed into your skin to put a drug or medicine into your body or to take out blood.

4. Specimen tube is a narrow container used to store specimen.

Task 5

1. tourniquet　　　　　　2. specimen tube　　　　　　3. cotton stick

Task 6

Setting 1:

1. I'm going to collect your urine to do a urinalysis.

2. It can indicate problems in kidneys.

3. I have brought you a urinal—this bottle.

4. Please pass urine into it.

5. I will use a disposable dipstick to make sure there is protein or blood in the urine specimen.

6. It only takes several minutes.

7. I will do the test in the ward.

8. The specimen won't be sent to the lab.

9. Please ring when it is ready.

Setting 2:

10. Next time you open your bowels we need to collect your stool to do a stool test.

11. It can indicate problems in the intestine.

12. Here is a stool collection tube with spoon on the lid.

13. Please get some of your stool with this little spoon and put it back into the tube.

14. Please avoid getting any other things into the tube.

15. Otherwise it might give us a false result.

16. Please ring when it is ready.

Dialogue Sample

Setting 1:

Nurse: Mr. Clinton, I'm going to collect your urine to do a urinalysis. It can indicate problems in kidneys.

Mr. Clinton: No problems. What do I need to do?

Nurse: I have brought you a urinal—this bottle. Please pass urine into it.

Mr. Clinton: In the bottle? May I know what it is testing for?

Nurse: I will use a disposable dipstick to make sure there is protein or blood in the urine specimen.

Mr. Clinton: Why will protein be in my urine?

Nurse: Protein will be found in urine when one gets kidney disease.

Mr. Clinton: Ok. How long can I know the result?

Nurse: It only takes several minutes. I will do the test in the ward. The specimen won't be sent to the lab.

Mr. Clinton: I see. I will give you now if you like.

Nurse: Thank you. Please ring when it is ready.

Setting 2:

Nurse: Mr. Blake, next time you open your bowels we need to collect your stool to do a stool test. It can indicate problems in the intestine.

Mr. Blake: Alright. What shall I do?

Nurse: Here is a stool collection tube with a spoon on the lid. Please get some of your stools with this little spoon and put it back into the tube. Then tighten the lid.

Mr. Blake: With this little spoon?

Nurse: Yes. Please avoid getting any other things into the tube, otherwise it might give us a false result.

Mr. Blake: Sure.

Nurse: Please ring when it is ready.

Part Three

Task 7

1. Complete blood count.

2. Blood.

3. 14: 05 on 7 November, 2018.

4. 16: 52 on 7 November, 2018.

5. Yes. Eric Naidu got increased leukocyte and neutrophil in his CBC report.

Task 8

Patient 1:	B	Patient 2:	A	Patient 3:	C

Task 9

Inter-professional English	Laypersons' English	Chinese
sputum	phlegm	痰
frequency	I pee more often than usual.	尿频
dysuria	It's painful when I pee.	排尿困难
urge incontinence	As soon as I get the urge to pee I must go.	尿急
loosely formed stool	soft/watery stool	大便未成形

More Practice

Sample:

Nurse: Good afternoon Mrs. Nelson. From your description of your symptoms, we suspect you have urinary tract infection. To confirm it, we need to get a midstream specimen of your urine. I have got a sterile specimen container and some disposable wipes for you.

Patient: OK. What shall I do?

Nurse: First please wash your hands thoroughly and clean the area around your urethra with these disposable wipes. So what's the step one?

Patient: Er… wash my hands and clean the area around my urethra?

Nurse: Yes. Then take the lid off and don't touch the inside of the container. Otherwise the specimen will be contaminated by bacteria. Do you get my point?

Patient: You mean I should avoid contamination from bacteria on my hands. Take the lid off without touching the inside.

Nurse: After that, you pass some urine into the toilet for a few second. Then urinate into this specimen container until it's about a quarter to a half full. That's the middle part of the stream of urine. Do you see what I mean?

Patient: I think so. Let me repeat it. I pass some urine into the toilet then some more into the container.

Nurse: That's exactly what I want you to do. Last but not least, tighten the lid and pass it to me, please.

Patient: Ok. That's quite important, isn't it?

Nurse: You are right. It's important to keep the specimen from contamination, otherwise we will get a false reading. Is that explanation clear? Do you have any questions?

Patient: No, thanks. I will do as you said.

Nurse: Ok. Please ring when it is ready.

Unit 5

Communication Focus

1. Because pain assessment is critical to optimal pain management interventions. While pain is a highly subjective experience, its management necessitates objective standards of care. The nurse should use various questions which can reflect the patient's subjective feeling without interference of their opinions.

2. A is better. When patients express or voice their physical pain, as a nurse, you need to reassure the patients that you have actually heard the complaint and can empathize with them. The promptness of your response to their requests for analgesia or to be seen by a doctor, are the practical manifestations of your concern.

Part One

Task 1

1. aching	2. stabbing	3. sharp	4. tingling
5. burning	6. throbbing	7. tender	8. shooting
9. dull	10. colicky		

Task 2

a. Conversation 4   b. Conversation 1   c. Conversation 3

d. Conversation 5   e. Conversation 2   f. Conversation 6

Task 3

Patient	Type of Pain	Body Part Involved
1	aching pain	arms
2	stabbing pain	backside
3	sharp pain	back
4	tingling pain	extremities
5	burning pain	stomach

Patient	Type of Pain	Body Part Involved
6	throbbing pain	right side of the head
7	tender pain	tummy
8	shooting pain	right lower abdomen
9	dull pain	chest
10	colicky pain	abdomen

Part Two

Task 4

A

1. no pain   2. mild pain   3. moderate pain

4. severe pain   5. very severe pain   6. unbearable pain

B

1. d   2. a   3. h   4. k   5. f   6. l   7. b   8. c   9. i   10. e   11. g   12. j

Task 5

Pain A

1. left shoulder   2. five   3. sharp pain

4. moving or getting out of bed   5. painkillers and heat packs

Pain B

1. right leg   2. four   3. burning pain

4. changing the dressing   5. non-stick dressings/pain relievers

Pain C

1. lower back   2. nine   3. aching pain

4. moving or sitting in the chair   5. analgesia/painkillers

Task 6

Sample

(N=nurse; P=patient)

N: Hello, Mr. Mc Garr. My name is Jenny. I'm taking care of you today.

P: Hello, Jenny. Nice to meet you.

N: How do you feel today?

P: I'm not very well today. I've got a lot of pain.

N: Oh, dear, I'm sorry to hear that. I've brought a pain chart so you can explain your pain a bit better.

P: Er, it's fine.

N: Where's the pain, Mr. Mc Garr?

P: There are two areas which hurt.

N: OK. Can you tell me on a scale of zero to ten what is the worst pain you've had in the last twenty-four hours in each area?

P: OK.

N: Can you show me the first one on the picture of the body?

P: It's around my liver.

N: OK. What's the pain in your liver like?

P: It's aching pain.

N: What sets the pain off?

P: It starts when I get out of bed to walk around.

N: How strong is the pain right now?

P: Er, a five. I had to get back to bed because of the pain.

N: OK, I'll label that pain "A". What makes the pain better?

P: The painkillers help a lot.

N: OK. What about the next one?

P: The wound in the right leg.

N: OK. That's "B". What starts the pain in your right leg?

P: It only hurts when the nurse changes the dressing.

N: What's the pain like?

P: It's sharp pain—around an eight out of ten.

N: What helps the pain?

P: Those non-stick dressings are good. And I have some pain relievers before the nurse does the dressing.

Part Three

Task 7

1. acupuncture	2. hypnotherapy	3. massage	4. aromatherapy
5. analgesia	6. hydrotherapy	7. heat pack	8. music therapy
9. chiropractic therapy	10. herbal therapy		

Task 8

a. example 4	b. example 1	c. example 5
d. example 2	e. example 6	f. example 3

Task 9

Sample:

OK, now we are up to Jim Sullivan in bed 3. Jim was admitted today for palliative care and pain control. He's got cancer of the liver. He was in quite a lot of pain when he first arrived. He had pain in the liver area and he described this as an aching pain. Jim was taking regular analgesia at home but it's not enough now. He rated the pain as 9 out of 10 when I spoke to him. Doctor Donnely saw Jim this morning and ordered a syringe driver. I explained to Jim that this would give him a small amount of painkiller medication continuously. He also finds that a heat pack on his back helps a lot.

More Practice

Sample:

(N=nurse; P=patient)

N: Hello, Charles. My name is Jenny. I'm taking care of you today.

P: Hello, Jenny. Nice to meet you.

N: How do you feel today?

P: I'm not very well today. I've got a lot of pain.

N: I'm sorry to hear that. Can you tell me where the pain is?

P: I've been having some pain in my joints, especially the knees.

N: How long have you been having the pain?

P: I'd say it started three or four months ago. It's been getting worse recently.

N: Are you having any other problems like weakness, fatigue or headaches?

P: Well, I've certainly felt under the weather.

N: How strong is the pain exactly? On a scale of one to ten, how would you describe the intensity of the pain?

P: Well, I'd say the pain is about an eight on a scale of one to ten. Like I said, it's really bad. It keeps coming back...

N: Is there anything which seems to make pain worse?

P: It gets worse when I stand up and put the weight on my knees. And nothing seems to help me to relieve pain.

N: It seems you have some inflammation in your knees.

P: That's a relief.

N: Your doctor has prescribed ibuprofen and the swelling will go down. And you can also put some heat packs on the knees when you are painful. You'll feel better after that.

P: OK. Thanks.

Unit 6

Communication Focus

1. When you address a patient, frequently use their names. Ideally use their first name, but only if they have given you the permission to do so.

2. Topics may include their work, family, pastimes or anything else that interests them. Of course, some patients might not feel like conversing and if you sense that is the case, then give them the space they need.

Part One

Task 1

a. capsule   b. ointment   c. solution   d. suppository   e. powder   f. tablet

g. inhaler   h. syrup   i. spray   j. drop   k. injection

Task 2

1. d	2. g	3. e	4. f	5. a	6. c	7. b
8. h	9. i	10. n	11. j	12. k	13. l	14. m

Task 3

1. 10 milligrams; by mouth; 90 days

2. 40 milligrams; three times a day; before meals/after meals

3. 20 milligrams; twice a day

Part Two

Task 4

1. g	2. a	3. j	4. h	5. b
6. f	7. c	8. i	9. d	10. e

Task 5

1. on an empty stomach

2. rinse your mouth with water

3. shake the bottle

4. discard the contents after this date

5. in the fridge

6. avoid too much sun

Task 6

1. Don't forget to keep the insulin in the fridge.

2. It's important that you shake the bottle before taking syrup.

3. Make sure you take antibiotics on an empty stomach.

4. Remember to rinse your mouth with water after you use inhaler.

5. You must complete the course of medication to get the optimized effect.

Part Three

Task 7

The right patient:	Check the patient's full name by checking the hospital label on the Prescription Chart and by checking the patient's identity bracelet; also check the patient's date of birth if necessary
The right medication:	Crosscheck the name of the medication on the Prescription Chart and the medication label
The right dose:	Crosscheck the dose of the medication on the Prescription Chart and the medication label
The right route:	Check the route of medication on the Prescription Chart
The right time:	Check how often the medication is to be given and at what time

Task 8

The right drug

The right patient

The right route

The right dose

The right time

Task 9

Sample

Nurse A: Susan, are you busy at the moment? Would you mind checking the medication for my patient with me now?

Nurse B: No, I am available now.

Nurse A: Right. It's for Mr. Zelnic in bed 1. Here's his Medication Chart.

Nurse B: Let me see. Mr. Zelnic, yes, and bed 1, yes. What's the medication you need to check?

Nurse A: I need you to check his anticoagulant medication. He's on warfarin at the moment.

Nurse B: Mm, warfarin. Yeah, that's what's written here.

Nurse A: And he's taking it orally.

Nurse B: Per os, yes, that's correct. What time is it due?

Nurse A: It's due at sixteen hundred hours, so that's now.

Nurse B: Sixteen hundred hours. Correct. We just need to check his INR before we give it, don't we? What was his INR result today?

Nurse A: His INR's down to one point five. Ideally, the doctors want it to be between two and two point five. Until it gets up to that level, he'll be taking 5mg of warfarin; then it can be reduced.

Nurse B: Yeah, poor guy. He's been really sick, hasn't he?

Nurse A: Yeah, he has. All right, here's the bottle of warfarin 5mg. Can you see the label to check the dose?

Nurse B: Yeah, I can. Um, it's warfarin 5mg.

Nurse A: I'm taking out one tablet.

Nurse B: Yep, one tablet.

Nurse A: I'll sign the medication chart first. There we are.

Nurse B: OK, let me counter sign for you. Right, that's done.

Nurse A: Thanks. I'll go and give it to him now. Thanks for your help.

More Practice

Sample:

Nurse: Hi, how are you feeling now?

Joan: I'm not well. I've gotten a splitting head.

Nurse: I'm sorry to hear that. The physician has ordered some painkiller for you. I'm going to check some details before giving it to you. Is that OK?

Joan: Fine, many thanks.

Nurse: Can you tell me your full name?

Joan: Joan Mitchell.

Nurse: OK, it is correct on the medication chart. Do you mind if I check your ID bracelet?

Joan: Fine, it's on my left wrist.

Nurse: I'll crosscheck the information on the medication chart and your ID bracelet.

Joan: Oh, my God. It's too complicated.

Nurse: It can assure the safety for you. Now, I'll check the medicine. The name of medicine is Demerol, right. The dose is 75mg. Yes, it's correct on the label. And you will take it by mouth.

Joan: So, one tablet, by mouth. What's that for?

Nurse: Right. It can help you ease your pain. Here is some tepid water.

Joan: I hope it will work soon. I can't bear the pain anymore.

Nurse: Don't worry. I'll inform the doctor if it is not relieved.

Joan: And when will I get another tablet?

Nurse: After three hours, you can have another one.

Joan: OK, fantastic! I want to have a sleep. Can you turn off the light?

Nurse: OK. Press the button if you need some help.

Joan: You are so considerable. See you.

Unit 7

Communication Focus

1. Non-verbal communication often speaks much louder than verbal communication, not just in Western culture, but in Asian culture too. Therefore, in WNES (Western native English speaking) countries, healthcare nurses become aware that it is crucial that they are sending exact non-verbal signals or body language to patients and other colleagues. Patients are often in very vulnerable and sensitive states of mind throughout their hospitalization and sometimes the nurse only needs to make the slightest unintentional slip, such as avoiding eye contact, and the therapeutic patient-nurse relationship might be seriously compromised.

2. a. Eye contact is essential. You should focus closely on your patients or colleagues when they are speaking. However, you can occasionally look away when you speak.

   b. Facial expression needs to be appropriate to the situation and generally it should demonstrate interest and concern.

   c. Smiling is a really important way of conveying approval, interest, encouragement or humour. Don't hesitate to smile whenever you see your patients or colleagues.

   d. Your posture needs to be relaxed in appearance and you should face the person you are communicating with.

   e. Physical proximity should be optimum, i.e. neither stand too far away from nor too close to the other person.

   f. Tone of voice can often be a more important signal of the nurses' real feelings than their actual verbal content, so send relaxing communication signals to your patient by speaking to them in a calm, gentle voice that isn't too fast.

Part One

Task 1

1. d	2. g	3. e	4. c	5. h
6. a	7. j	8. i	9. b	10. f

Task 2

1. IV pole   2. IV solution   3. IV line

4. IV infusion pump   5. IV cannula   6. fluid balance chart

Task 3

		Fluid Type	Volume Infused	Drip Rate Calculator	Date/Time	Concentration Percentage
1	1000 ml		√			
2	30/5 11:00				√	
3	500ml/hr			√		
4	167 DPM			√		
5	5%					√
6	Normal Saline	√				

Part Two

Task 4

1. Check the IV solution against the physician's orders.

2. Wash hands thoroughly before inserting an IV.

3. Use the sterile technique when inserting an IV line.

4. Prime the IV tubing to remove air from the system.

5. Label the tubing, and the solution bags clearly, indicating the date and time when changed.

Task 5

N: Good morning, Ms. Smith. It's time to give you intravenous infusion.

P: Excuse me, could you tell me about the use of the intravenous fluid?

N: Of course. The fluid can provide energy for you and prevent you from electrolytic imbalances after the operation.

(*IV infusion is set up.*)

P: Would you please let the fluid drop more quickly?

N: Your intravenous fluid must be given slowly so as not to overload you.

P: Is it possible for my sister to stay here with me?

N: Yes, of course. But I don't think it is necessary. Your condition isn't that serious.

P: Oh, I see.

N: Is there anything I can do for you?

P: I feel a little cold. Could you help me adjust the air conditioner?

N: Please wait a moment. Do you want another blanket?

P: No, thanks.

N: Just press the button if you need any help.

P: Thank you. Sorry to bother you.

N: You are welcome.

Task 6

1. c	2. f	3. i	4. e	5. g
6. b	7. h	8. d	9. a	

Part Three

Task 7

1. 03:00	2. 11:00	3. 1000ml	4. 30/05
5. IV	6. 5%	7. 100ml	8. K.B

Task 8

Dr. Harris;

Resite cannula Mrs. Blake;

Michael to call Dr. Harris regarding when cannula needs resite;

Due time next IV ABs;

Bleep Dr. Harris 467

Task 9

Sample:

(J=Jane Smith, nurse; R=Rose Williams, ward nurse)

J: Good morning, Ward 16C Jane Smith speaking.

R: Hello, it's Rose Williams here. I'm the nurse of the IV Infusion Room. I'm calling to tell you that Mr. Henry in your ward is booked to have a PICC line inserted at 10:30 a.m. tomorrow. Can I speak to the nurse looking after him?

J: Oh, Lucy's looking after Mr. Henry today. She's just on a break. Can I take a message for her?

R: Yeah. Could you please tell Lucy that a porter is needed to bring Mr. Henry to the IV Infusion Room and don't forget to take the IV Prescription Chart with him.

J: OK. Let me just read that message back to you. You want Lucy to take Mr. Henry to have a PICC line inserted at 10:30 a. m. tomorrow. And she should book a porter to take Mr. Henry to the IV Infusion Room and the IV Prescription Chart should be taken with him.

R: That's right.

J: OK. I'll make sure I pass your message on to Lucy.

R: Thanks, Jane.

J: You are welcome.

Date of message	18/10/2018
Time of message	10.00 hrs
Name of caller	Rose Williams, nurse
Nature of call	to have a PICC line inserted, to Mr. Henry
Instructions	1. have a PICC line inserted tomorrow 10: 30 a.m.
	2. need a porter to bring Mr. Henry to the IV Infusion Room
	3. take the IV Prescription Chart
Message documented in Patient Record	Yes/Not necessary
Signature of call recipient	Jane Smith

More Practice

Sample:

(N=nurse; P=patient)

N: Good morning, Ms. Sara Young. It's time to give you intravenous infusion.

P: Sorry, I don't need the medication by infusion anymore.

N: Why is that?

P: Well, I have been receiving the drug by infusion over a number of weeks. And my physician Mr. Black has agreed to change the mode of administration from IV to oral.

N: Oh, please don't be worried, Ms. Sara Young. You know, we must strictly follow the physician's order. I'll check the order sheet and speak with Mr. Black to see whether your order should be changed today. Anyway, don't worry, and take it easy, OK?

P: OK, it doesn't matter. Thank you.

N: You are welcome.

Unit 8

Communication Focus

1. You should always first check the policy in your workplace. If the patient agrees to disclose information about his/her clinical progress, then you can generally proceed to do so.

If your patient is physically or mentally incapable of giving a legally valid consent, then you need to ask his family members for permission. If not, you are likely to end up in court.

Obviously, you can also communicate about your patients with fellow health professionals who are employed in your hospital and are also involved in the patient's clinical care. Catering staff or cleaners should not know the patient's information unless it directly relates to their jobs. For example, the catering staff that delivers meals to a patient may need to know that he/she is diabetic, but doesn't need to know what medications he/she is taking for the diabetes or any other confidential clinical information. Cleaners, of course, may need to be informed of specific infectious hazards that patients may encounter.

2. a. When talking to the patients about their medical history and the current condition, ensure that you do so discreetly. You may need to speak softly, close the bedside curtains and, even find another private room if practical.

   b. If you suspect that something you might discuss with the patient is a highly sensitive matter, e.g. issues relating to sex, violence, death, drug dependence or mental illness, then you should ask the patients if they would prefer to talk in a more private setting.

   c. Considerations a & b above also apply to patients' family members and friends.

   d. Whatever you do, don't discuss one patient's condition in any detail with other patients. This not only is disregarding the patient's privacy, but may also breach his/her legal rights to confidentiality.

   e. In some Western countries, people can find nakedness or even partial nakedness extremely embarrassing, so pay great attention to maintaining the patient's privacy to protect their dignity. Whenever the patient is not covered properly with clothing, make sure that bedside curtains are drawn and doors are closed etc. Obviously, this applies to when a patient is being showered or toileted, too.

Part One

Task 1

1. washbasin	2. towel	3. toothbrush	4. gloves
5. brush	6. shampoo	7. detergent	8. clinical disposable bag
9. sink	10. toothpaste	11. bucket	12. razor
13. kidney basin	14. shaving cream	15. pyjamas	16. paper towels
17. blanket	18. bin	19. swab	20. soap

Task 2

1. inspection	2. hygiene	3. spillage	4. fluid	5. urine
6. staff	7. considerate	8. swab	9. sponge	10. mouth wash

Task 3

1. 2; 10
2. regularly cleaned
3. between patients
4. every three hours; twice
5. every two hours; once a day
6. the average time
7. before putting on gloves and after removing gloves
8. short-staffed

Part Two

Task 4

1. cleanse the body of all dirt, sweat, germs and other things
2. There are three different types of baths

3. a complete bed bath, a partial bath, and a tub or shower bath

4. with the bed bath, shower or tub bath; more often

5. once a day or once every couple of days; their underarms and legs

6. brushing the teeth, flossing the teeth, and rinsing the mouth; dentures

7. skin breakdown, corns, bleeding, broken, chipped or absent nails, as well as blue or pale nail beds

8. with shampoo and conditioner

9. comb or brush their hair a couple of times a day

10. infection; injuries

Task 5

1. Yes, very well.

2. There are some small ulcers.

3. It is mainly to prevent bedsores.

4. Because the clothes are all wet from sweating during the night.

5. No, he doesn't.

Task 6

1. oral care	2. back massage	3. personal hygiene
4. at the bedside	5. seated near the sink	6. parts of their bodies
7. complete bed bath	8. massaging back	9. bed linens or clothing
10. positioning patients		

Part Three

Task 7

1. 枕骨	2. 肩胛骨	3. 肘部	4. 骶骨	5. 脚后跟
6. 脚趾	7. 大腿；股	8. 股骨粗隆	9. 小腿；胫	10. 肱骨上端
11. 胸腔	12. 膝盖骨			

Task 8

1. 15 minutes	2. once every two hours	3. discoloration
4. more likely to occur	5. delicate	6. healthy and nutritious
7. hygiene practices	8. activity	9. quits smoking
10. reduce pressure	11. moist	12. dry
13. infection	14. damaged tissues	

Task 9

Sample:

Nurse: Good morning, Mr. Black. Did you have a good night?

Mr. Black: Not very good. It was too hot.

Nurse: Let me help you to clean up and make you comfortable.

Mr. Black: Thank you very much.

Nurse: Please turn over to the other side. I'll rub your back with a hot towel and then massage it with alcohol and talcum powder.

Mr. Black: Why do you do that?

Nurse: It's mainly to stimulate your blood circulation to prevent bedsores.

Mr. Black: Oh, I see. My clothes are all wet from sweating during the night.

Nurse: I'll help you to change at once.

Mr. Black: Good.

Nurse: I'm also going to change the sheets on your bed.

Mr. Black: Should I get out of the bed?

Nurse: No, you needn't. I can do the change without your getting out of the bed. (*After changing*) Are you feeling comfortable now?

Mr. Black: Oh, yes. I'm feeling better now. Thank you so much.

More Practice

Sample:

(N=nurse; P=patient)

N: How are you feeling, Mrs. White?

P: I've got a pain on my shoulder.

N: Yeah, because there is an ulcer there.

P: Why is that so?

N: Well, just because you sit in the chair too long.

P: Is it serious?

N: Don't worry. The reddened area is only 4 cm. And it doesn't blanch to pressure. It is just Stage I ulcer. So it's not that serious.

P: So will you do something for it?

N: Surely. We'll promote healing through removing the pressure, protecting the wound from contamination.

P: (*Points to one piece of equipment*) What's it for?

N: It is a pressure-relieving equipment. We'll use it to help you to reduce the pressure on your shoulder.

P: Does it work well?

N: We've already checked it. It is working effectively.

P: Will it cause much pain?

N: Surely not. After reducing the pressure, we also make sure that the reddened area is protected from moisture damage. You'll be all right soon. But you'd better change position every 15 minutes when you sit in the chair.

P: I see. Thank you.

Unit 9

Communication Focus

1. Open-ended questions are those that are less likely to be answered with a simple "yes" or "no".

2. Because those open-ended questions invite the person being questioned to give some kinds

of descriptive answers relating to their medical condition or mental/emotional state.

3. In healthcare communication, both types of questions are extremely useful. Using closed questions is like ticking off each item, while open-ended questioning can sometimes elicit more detailed and accurate responses from patients. When taking a patient's history, you are more likely to miss out on obtaining vital information when overusing closed questions.

Part One

Task 1

Category	Food Item
Good source of protein	tuna fish pie, cheese pizza, lentil soup, roast beef, fried eggs, baked beans, burgers, lamb kebab
Good source of carbohydrate	egg noodles, cheese pizza, fried rice, boiled potatoes, doughnut
Dairy product	cheese pizza, chocolate pudding (if made with milk), yoghurt, milk
High in fat	cheese pizza, grilled burgers, fried eggs, lamb kebab, fried onion rings, doughnut, chocolate pudding, fried rice
High in vitamin C	orange juice, steamed broccoli
Low in vitamin	doughnut, fried onion rings
Junk food	doughnut, burgers, fried onion rings
High in caloriy	doughnut, cheese pizza, chocolate pudding
Way of cooking food	grill, roast, fry, boil, bake, stir-fry, steam

Task 2

1. sugar	2. protein	3. dairy	4. fats	5. health
6. vitamin	7. mineral	8. energy	9. calcium	10. carbohydrate

Task 3

1. energy	2. fuel	3. bones	4. blood	5. fight
6. repair	7. skin	8. digest		

Part Two

Task 4

Diet restrictions and requirements	(√) yes ( ) no	If YES **to gain some weight**
a) BMI **17.9**		
b) Food allergies	(√) yes ( ) no	If YES **peanuts**
c) Last meal (date/time) **at 10: 00 last night**	Give details	**a bowl of soup , some toast, and etc.**

1. slightly underweight	2. gain weight
3. normal weight	4. doesn't eat enough

Task 5

1. What kind of diet do you recommend for me?

2. Some patients find it helpful to eat small meals five or six times a day.

3. How has your appetite been lately?

4. Your body needs the nutrition so that you can regain your strength and energy.

5. Excess weight is associated with an increased risk of heart disease.

6. You should avoid fatty meat and fried foods in order to prevent high blood cholesterol.

Task 6

Sample:

N: Would you mind telling me what your weight is?

P: Two hundred and eleven pounds.

N: Your height, please?

P: I'm five feet six inches tall. How severe is my weight problem?

N: Generally, a patient with a body mass index, or BMI(Body Mass Index) of 25 to 29.9 is considered overweight; one with a BMI of 30 or higher is considered obese. And yours is 34.1. I'm afraid it's a little serious.

P: Without intervention, what should I expect?

N: Excess weight is associated with an increased risk of heart disease, stroke, high blood pressure, diabetes, gallstones and some forms of cancer.

P: How much weight should I lose?

N: Permanent weight loss is extraordinarily difficult, studies show, and ideal weights are rarely reached. A weight loss goal should be realistic, researchers say, and you should also take into account your family history and current risk factors. Many people find it useful to set goals in stages — for example, to lose 10 pounds within two months, then another 10, and so forth.

P: What kind of diet do you recommend for me?

N: Avoid diets that exclude the entire categories of food. Popular high-protein menus may work for some patients in the short term, some researchers have found, but fruits and vegetables should be the foundation of any long-term diet.

P: Does meal frequency matter?

N: Some patients find it helpful to eat small meals five or six times a day. Complicated regimens involving macronutrients consumed only at certain time of the day have not been well supported by research.

P: Thank you for your advice.

Part Three

Task 7

1. glucose	2. hormone	3. cure	4. borderline	5. gestational

Task 8

1. a   2. a   3. a   4. b   5. d

Task 9

1. Are there any members in your family who have diabetes

2. diabetic

3. insulin therapy

4. Could you tell me something about the diabetic diet

5. sugar and sweets

6. What else should I know

7. blood and urine

8. do some exercises

More Practice

Sample:

Nurse: Good morning, Mr. Black.

Mr. Black: Good morning.

Nurse: How are you feeling?

Mr. Black: Not bad. I was told I'm underweight. Is it serious?

Nurse: Well, it's not good for people, since it will cause nutritional deficiencies, weakened immune system, and it'll also cause fertility problems.

Mr. Black: So I belong to the first case, right?

Nurse: Yeah. You're lacking nutrients that your body needs to work properly, such as calcium, iron, vitamins etc. Calcium, for example, is important for the maintenance of strong and healthy bones. If you don't get enough calcium, you risk developing osteoporosis (fragile bone disease) in later life. If you're not consuming enough iron, you may develop anaemia, which can leave you feeling drained and tired.

Mr. Black: Oh, I see, but I'm in an intensive exercise program. How can I put on weight safely?

Nurse: You should try to choose a variety of different foods from the five main food groups, learn more about these food groups and how they form part of a healthy diet, and base your diet on the Eat-Well Guide.

Mr. Black: Ok. And then?

Nurse: And try to avoid relying on high-calorie foods full of saturated fat and sugar—such as chocolate, cakes and sugary drinks—to gain weight. These foods can increase body fat instead of decreasing body mass and increase your risk of developing high levels of cholesterol in your blood. Therefore, aim for regular meals and occasional snacks.

Mr. Black: Sorry, I don't think I really understand.

Nurse: Well, that means you need to avoid fatty meat and fried foods in order to prevent high blood cholesterol and you need to eat enough fruits and vegetables every day. Choose Whole grain food if possible such as potatoes, bread, rice, pasta or other starchy carbohydrates.

Mr. Black: And?

Nurse: And have some dairy or dairy alternatives, choose lower-fat and lower-sugar options, and eat some beans, pulses, fish, eggs, meat and other food rich in protein. Have two portions of fish every week – one of which should be oily, such as salmon or mackerel, and choose unsaturated oils and spreads, such as sunflower or rapeseed, having them in small amounts.

Mr. Black: Anything else?

Nurse: Yeah. You should also drink plenty of fluids, 6-8 cups/glasses a day, but try not to have drinks just before meals to avoid feeling too full to eat.

Mr. Black: Got it.

Nurse: Don't worry. You'll recover soon if you follow the doctor's advice.

Mr. Black: I'm sure I will.

Unit 10

Communication Focus

1. a. Accept the patient's feelings and don't be afraid to say "I can really understand that you feel this way".

b. Never get into an argument about the logicality of the patient's feelings.

c. If the patient is a bit awkward about expressing his/her feelings, then help him/her by saying, "I imagine you feel quite sad about this, it's totally natural to feel that way in your situation. I've certainly got time to listen to you if you want to talk about it."

d. Send warm, friendly and accepting cues such as good eye contact, a concerned facial expression, occasional and gentle smiles when appropriate, and an open and relaxed posture. …

2. Spend time explaining what happens in the pre-op and post-op periods so it is more familiar to your patient. Ensure that you have uninterrupted time to discuss any concerns with your patient so that he/she may feel comfortable talking about them. Be aware of cultural or language factors which may cause more anxiety and ensure an interpreter is at hand if necessary.

3. Strategies useful for a child: allow the child to touch equipment, for example, oxygen masks; reassure the child that a parent will accompany him/her to the operating theatre; allow the child to take a special toy with him/her or keep the toy to wait for him/her.

Part One

Task 1

1. operation	2. signature	3. anaesthetist	4. antiseptic
5. interfere	6. fluid	7. muscle	8. enema

Task 2

1. I'm going to	2. I'll	3. you'll	4. Will
5. I'm going to	6. won't; will	7. I'll; You'll	

Task 3

1. Mrs. Wiseman has to wash twice with antiseptic wash, one in the evening before the operation and the other on the morning of the operation. She also has to remove her nail polish.

2. Because there is a choking risk with anaesthesia.

3. To prevent DVTs.

Part Two

Task 4

| 1. c | 2. a | 3. e | 4. b | 5. f | 6. d |

Task 5

1. He is very nervous.

2. Keyhole surgery, which is also called minimally invasive surgery.

3. A gastroscope.

4. The surgery is performed through the throat into the stomach, so there won't be a puncture on surface.

5. Because he'll have a general anaesthesia that makes him feel nothing during the surgery.

6. Until his swallow reflex and the bowels are working again.

7. Soon after returning to the ward, when Mr. Kim thinks he can pass urine.

Task 6

| a. 4 | b. 1 | c. 3 | d. 5 | e. 1 | f. 4 |

(open)

Part Three

Task 7

1. YES	2. YES	3. YES	4. YES	5. NO or N/A
6. NO or N/A	7. NO or N/A	8. NO or N/A	9. NO or N/A	10. YES
11. YES	12. NO or N/A	13. YES	14. YES	

Urine last voided at 10: 20 a.m.

Catheterized N/A

Fluid last given at 11:00 p.m.

Food last given at 6:00 p.m.

Task 8

1. ID bracelet

2. Consent form signed

14. Pre-med given and signed for

Task 9

| a. 4 | b. 10 | c. 8 | d. 3 | e. 1 |
| f. 6 | g. 2 | h. 9 | i. 7 | j. 5 |

More Practice

Sample:

(N=nurse; P=patient)

N: Hello, David. How are you feeling?

P: I feel OK, but I'm very nervous.

N: Are you? What's worrying you?

P: Well, I'm worried that the anaesthetic won't be strong enough, and I'll be in pain, but won't be able to speak.

N: Don't worry about that. If you like, I'll ask the anaesthetist to explain exactly what he does.

P: Thanks. That would help.

N: In a moment I'm going to give you a pre-med. That'll make you feel nice and relaxed and sleepy.

P: OK.

N: After that we'll take you through to the theatre, and the anaesthetist will connect you up to the monitoring equipment. Then he'll give you some drugs that'll send you to sleep.

P: How will I feel when I wake up?

N: You may feel a little sick or you might be really hungry. We'll give you pain relief while you're waking up, and then when you're fully awake, you'll have a little pump—I've got one here (we call it PCA)—which you control by yourself.

P: How will I know when to use it?

N: When you feel pain, you just press the button. Here, have a try.

P: OK. So I won't have any pain at all then?

N: Well, you'll just feel very mild pain if you use the pump.

P: That doesn't sound too bad.

Unit 11

Communication Focus

1. A patient's autonomy is his/her right to decide what action will or won't be taken in order to treat his/her health problems. This right is protected by related laws. In most cases, patients can refuse medical treatment at any time. A patient's independence should be promoted as much as possible. Now patients are encouraged to do things for themselves and get out of bed as soon as medically possible. This approach can not only speed up recovery and lessen hospitalization days, but also enhance self-confidence in them. At the same time, nursing workloads are greatly reduced. Thus, nurses are able to improve the quality of care.

2. In communication with patients, nurses should not criticize or ignore a patient's decision even if they consider it to be a bad one. They should explain the pros and cons of each possible treatment option to the patient and let him/her make the decision for himself/herself. Indeed, a patient should be made to feel in charge of his/her situation as much as possible instead of seeing himself/herself as a passive object. For example, when the patient is present, staff should generally talk with

him/her and make him/her feel like having has the right to speak in what is going on. Another example is to ensure you say "please" when requesting the patient to do something and say "thank you" once he/she has complied. It is a powerful message that you respect the patient's autonomy: his/her right to say "yes" or "no" to anything you request of him/her.

Part One

Task 1

1. splenectomy	2. therapy	3. pethidine
4. dextrose	5. analgesia	6. complication

Task 2

1. a	2. e	3. c	4. b	5. d

Task 3

2. 13/15	3. 36°C	4. 72	5. 97	6. dextrose
7. patent	8. Clips	9. NAD	10. 75	11. oral
12. redivac	13. intact			

Part Two

Task 4

1. hypothermia	2. groggy	3. anaesthetic
4. reaction	5. sensation	

Task 5

1. c	2. e	3. h	4. g
5. b	6. d	7. f	8. a

Task 6

Sample:

(N=nurse; P=patient)

P: I'm still feeling cold. Is that normal?

N: Yeah, it's OK. It's called hypothermia. It happens sometimes if the operation takes a long time. I'll get you an extra blanket to help warm you up.

P: I'm awake now, but I still feel a bit groggy.

N: That's because you've had an anesthetic. You'll feel better soon.

P: My throat feels really sore. It's hard to swallow.

N: Don't worry, that's normal. It's just caused by the tube they put down your throat during the surgery. I'll get you some ice chips to suck soon.

P: I feel like I'd be sick if I ate anything.

N: Nausea is sometimes a reaction to post-operative pain. I'll keep an eye on that.

P: I'm in bad pain, and everything hurts.

N: That's quite normal. Patients who've had abdominal surgery are often in quite a bit of discomfort. I'll get you an injection for the pain.

P: I feel like I can't move because it's going to be painful.

N: It's quite common to avoid any movement which might cause discomfort, but it's important that I help you to move around and change positions.

P: I feel as if I want to go to the toilet all the time.

N: It's quite usual to have that sensation, even though you've got a catheter in your bladder.

P: I feel dizzy, too. It's like I'm going to fall out of bed.

N: That's OK. It takes a little while to be orientated again after an anaesthetic. I'm going to put these bed rails up while you're feeling a bit wobbly and get you some pain relief. Here's the call bell if you need me.

Part Three

Task 7

1. bowel   2. rinse; spit   3. dizzy; light-headed

4. constipation; lung   5. edge; shoulder

Task 8

1. Not too great. He feels thirsty.

2. No, he can't. He asks for some painkillers.

3. He should have intravenous antibiotics three times a day.

More Practice

Sample:

(A=Ali, patient; N=nurse)

N: Hello, Ali. How are you feeling now?

A: Oh, not good. Everything hurts.

N: Mm, I can imagine. You've got lots of cuts and bruises. Can you tell me where the pains are?

A: Yeah. My head, my cheek…um, the broken cheek, I mean. My arms hurt where the cuts are and my chest hurts, too.

N: Can you tell me if the pain is the same all over or different?

A: I've got a throbbing headache, and my right cheek hurts when I touch it.

N: That's because you've got a broken cheek bone. The pain is referred to your head and you get a headache.

A: Oh. That makes sense.

N: What about the pain in your arms and chest?

A: It's a stinging pain in the shallow cuts, but this cut in my chest is quite deep, and the pain's like a knife.

N: When's the pain worse, John?

A: It's worse when I turn over or move.

N: OK, can you rate the pain for me? On a scale of zero to ten, zero is when you feel no pain and ten is when you feel the worst pain that you can imagine. What's the pain like now when you are at rest?

A: It's around six.

N: And when you move a bit?

A: It gets worse. Seven, at least.

N: All right, I'll get you something for the pain. Now, I notice you've been ordered paracetamol four hourly.

A: Yeah, I don't want it. It ain't strong enough.

N: No, not on its own, but the doctor ordered it for you because it works with the opioid painkillers to reduce the amount you need to take.

A: Er.

N: I mean, it reduces the number of injections you need to have by twenty to thirty percent. It's important to keep taking the paracetamol regularly.

A: Oh, I know. That's different then.

N: Is there anything else which relieves the pain?

A: One of the nurses gave me a heat pack for my chest, and that helped.

N: All right. I'll get the painkillers for you and try to put you in a comfortable position with some more pillows. I'll get a heat pack, too.

A: Thank you. I'll try to get some rest. It's hard to sleep when you're in pain.

N: Yes, it is. I'll pull the curtains around and dim the lights a bit for you as well. There you go.

Unit 12

Communication Focus

1. Safeguarding the patient's rights, with respect to his/her personal health information, is our ethical and legal obligation as healthcare providers. The nurse should promote, advocate and strive to protect the health, safety, and rights of the patient.

2. a. When the family members or the significant others are present with the patient, speak to them as well as the patient. Of course your focus should be on the patient, but frequent eye contact and inclusive body language should also be used with the family members.

   b. When doctors visit the patient, ensure that the family members are introduced to them and that they are included in all relevant meetings.

   c. Provide education and counseling to the family members as you do to the patient. If they are going to be assisting the patient after their discharge then they need to thoroughly understand all medications and pertinent healthcare information, too. Emotionally, they may also struggle in coping with the patient's health condition and need moral support and an opportunity to debrief.

Part One

Task 1

1. It's difficult for him/her to walk to the bathroom and pick things up.

2. Reading newspapers and magazines.

3. Doing exercises and nature walks.

4. He/She is considering whether he/she should go to a care home.

5. He/She is very lonely because his/her daughter lives in the USA.

6. He/She has a lot of problems. He/She is very deaf, without his/her hearing aid he/she hears nothing at all. He/She needs help getting dressed and getting in and out of the bath. He/She has a walking stick and he/she's very independent.

Task 2

a. hearing aid   b. dentures   c. grabber

d. glasses   e. walking frame   f. commode

1. c   2. f   3. e   4. b   5. a   6. d

Task 3

1. She likes nature and reading.

2. She has hearing problems and she doesn't have the patience to read the subtitles.

3. Two, one son and one daughter.

4. Her son lives in Australia, and her daughter lives in Canada. So she keeps in contact with them by email.

Part Two

Task 4

1. Devin   2. I see my family   3. Impolite or unfriendly people

4. Italian and Indian   5. eggs   6. wear

Task 5

1. tennis   2. cricket   3. classical   4. traditional

5. the big games   6. the news   7. don't really read 8. walking stick

9. walking frame   10. don't need   11. grabber   12. have no

13. have   14. glasses

Task 6

（答案合理即可。以下为参考答案）

1. Sandy/Dipak   2. I see my family/I'm by myself

3. Impolite or unfriendly people/Noisy places

4. Italian/Indian   5. apples/fish   6. reading books/watching TV

7. the news   8. music   9. walking stick/walking frame

10. grabber   11. the hearing aid   12. glasses

Part Three

Task 7

(1) a. (F)   b. (F)   c. (F)   d. (A)   e. (A)

     f. (F)   g. (A)   h. (A)   i. (F)   j. (F)

(2) Ideal care home:

    Facilities: garden; TV room; laundry room; dining room; computer room; library

    Activities: aromatherapy treatment; exercise program; day trip; nature walk

Task 8

Julie wants: respect/privacy/more stimulation/to go home/independence

Julie doesn't like: Barbara/bingo/coach trips/the food

Task 9

Memory: forgetting recent conversations or events; forgetting names; inability to recognize familiar people, objects or places; complete loss of memory

Behaviour: ranging from minor changes in abilities and behaviour at the early stage to getting easily upset or aggressive at the later stage

Speech: loss of speech

Walking: shuffling gait; confinement to bed or a wheelchair

Daily life: ranging from needing some help with ADLs at the middle stage to needing constant help with ADLs etc. at the later stage

More Practice

Sample:

(N=nurse; M=Mrs. Green)

N: Good afternoon, Mrs. Green, nice to meet you. My name's Angela. My team will be taking care of you during your stay at the hospital.

M: Nice to meet you, too.

N: Now, I'm just going to ask you some questions first so that we can get to know you better. Is that OK?

M: Yes, of course.

N: First question: what would you like us to call you?

M: I prefer people to call me Julie if that's OK.

N: Yes, of course. It's your first week here, Julie. How do you feel?

M: A little sad.

N: Yes? Can you tell me why?

M: I had been suffering from COPD for 3 years and the doctor said I had to have a long-term hospitalization this time. I don't want some young nurse telling me what I can and cannot do. I want children around me. So you see, I'm…I'm sorry.

N: It's OK. I understand it's difficult for you at the moment. I hope we can make it easier for you. We're going to try, anyway. So, when do you feel happy?

M: That's easy—when I spend time with my family.

N: And who are the children in the photo?

M: My grandchildren, Selina, and that's Peter.

N: Ah, they're beautiful! When did you last see your family?

M: My son and his wife are in Australia, so it has been some long time since the last time I saw them. I miss all of them.

N: We have a small computer room. It's a good idea to reserve some time to use the computer to keep in contact with them by email. It's more and more popular with the patients.

M: Really? I might do that, thanks. Internet access is fine.

N: You're welcome. You can have a rest now. Please let me know if you need any help.

Unit 13

Communication Focus

1. While listening, you are getting information to understand and learn better; listening is crucial to understand others' perspectives, thoughts and values of speech. Active listening is all the more necessary as a means for you to ensure that you have properly understood your patients.

2. Thoughtful mind, eyes to catch, alert ears, being quiet, still hands, firm feet and so on are important. Active listening is a highly active mental process. A simple analogy to explain this would be that when a patient is telling you about either his/her emotional or clinical situation, you use the information he/she gives you to create a precise mental "painting" of what he/she has said. You may often need to ask him/her questions to clarify what was said, much as an artist frequently looks at his subject and adjusts the painting with light brushwork to ensure that it is a faithful representation of the original image, or in your active listening case, the original meaning.

Part One

Task 1

1. c	2. d	3. a	4. e
5. g	6. h	7. b	8. f

Task 2

2. cesarean	2. pregnancy	3. uterus	4. womb
5. abdomen	6. dilatation	7. nauseated	8. high-risk

Task 3

1. blood flow; placenta	2. good position; engaged	3. contractions
4. cramps	5. cervix	6. delivered

Part Two

Task 4

1. My contractions are so close together.
2. Your cervix is fully dilated.
3. It's time to go to the delivery room.
4. Is there a cramp coming?
5. Open your mouth, and breathe quickly and shallowly.
6. When the next cramp comes, you can start pushing down.
7. The head has descended into the vagina.
8. I'm going to make a small surgical incision at the perineum so the delivery will be easier.

Task 5

1. effacement and dilation of cervix
2. expulsion of fetus
3. separation of placenta

4. physical recovery

Task 6

Sample:

(W=Wang Li, midwife; F=Fang Tong, nurse; M=Mary, patient)

W: Mary, your cervix is fully dilated; it's time to go to the delivery room. Fang Tong, please help her

F: OK. Mary, you can lean on me. Don't worry!

M: OK, but I feel so dizzy and weak.

W: That's normal. Just sit down on the bed here. Mary, is there a cramp coming? Let's wait until it passes. Open your mouth, Breathe quickly and shallowly. Did the pain go away?

M: I think so.

W: Then you can lie down. Move your buttocks towards the end, and put your feet in the stirrups. When the next cramp comes, you can start pushing down. Wait until you can't hold it any longer and then start pushing down, just like when you go to the toilet.

M: There's another cramp coming.

W: Take a deep breath and push! Push harder! Take another breath and push again! Once more!

F: Oh, I see the baby's crown.

W: Now, I'm going to make a small surgical incision at the perineum so delivery will be easier, and you shouldn't have any serious tears.

F: OK, the head is out! Just one more push and you're done!

W: Congratulations! You have a healthy baby girl! You did a great job!

M: Thank you for your help!

Part Three

Task 7

a

Task 8

1. c

　　The mother sits down and is relaxed, and puts the baby's face close to her breast. Let the baby's nose next to her nipple, and their bodies form a straight line (chest to chest, belly to belly, chin to breast), with mother's hand holding the baby's buttocks. This is one of the popular breastfeeding positions during the first few weeks of nursing, when you're getting comfortable with your new job. A breastfeeding pillow can help lift baby and support your elbows.

2. b

　　To do this one, you recline back about 45 degrees wherever you like to nurse—on the couch, in bed, or on a recliner—and the baby lies face down on top of your breast with his/her arms hugging your breast on both sides.

3. d

　　Of the breastfeeding positions, this one—also sometimes called a clutch hold—is often what the first moms want to learn. With the football hold, the baby is tucked under your arm off to the side (yep, like a football) and held with one arm while you support your breast with the other arm. If you're holding the baby on the right side, the baby will latch onto your right breast while you support it with your left hand.

4. a

For this in-bed breastfeeding position, lie down on your side with the baby facing you. (You can put a breastfeeding pillow or a roll-up towel behind the baby to support his/her back.) The baby is nursed from the breast that's resting on the bed.

Task 9

1. "Early sucking" means mother-infant skin contact and assists breastfeeding within half an hour after birth.

2. It can stimulate reflection and increase milk secretion.

3. Keep the baby sucking the mother's nipples and the mother will be stimulated.

4. It's the best natural nutrition for the baby. It is not only economic, simple and with proper temperature, but also helpful in increasing the baby's immune function, add the baby's anti-disease capability, and promote the growth of the baby's brain cells. At the same time, it can also help the mother's uterus recovery, reduce post-partum bleeding, and reduce the chances of breast and ovarian cancer. And it can promote the bonding between the mother and her baby.

More Practice

Sample:

(N=nurse; P=patient)

N: Mrs. Li, how do you feel after resting?

P: Much better, thanks. But now I am so confused, as my mom wants me to have caesarean birth, but my mother-in-law insists I should deliver normally. I don't know how to make the choice.

N: Mrs. Li, I can see from the data that you are healthy and your status for giving birth is also good. I think that you can get through the birth smoothly. So maybe you can choose natural childbirth.

P: Could you tell me more about the childbirth?

N: OK. Natural childbirth is safer and carries less risks for moms and their babies. Studies prove that infant and mother mortality rates are lower in natural births. Medications used during labour can have a variety of negative effects on baby including lowered heart rate, difficulty in breathing and lowered breastfeeding success after delivery. Babies born naturally without medication are statistically more alert, responsive and have higher Apgar scores.

P: Alright, I see. It sounds it's better to choose natural childbirth. But I am very afraid of giving birth. Giving birth can be very painful, right?

N: At the beginning, you will feel a little pain during uterus contractions and cervix dilation. As the baby moves into the birth canal, labour is much easier to endure when you can use gravity to your benefit. One of the best ways to maximize your ability to labour naturally is by hiring a birth doula to assist you. She will support you during your labour by offering natural solutions for pain relief such as massage, meditation, water therapy, breathing techniques, positioning, moaning and hypnosis.

P: Oh, when my husband comes here later, we will discuss it. Thanks for your introduction.

N: Good. When you have made a decision, please tell me.

Unit 14

Communication Focus

1. Because when hospitalized patients feel anxious about their illness process, they may lose confidence in their own strengths or the positive recovery gains. Praising could remind them of these facts.

2. You did a good job. / Fabulous. / Good job. / You can do it. / You're improving. / You are on target…

Part One

Task 1

1. c   2. a   3. b

Task 2

1. occupational	2. therapy	3. treatment	4. physiotherapy
5. joint	6. muscle	7. nerve	8. massage

Task 3

1. Explain   2. benefits   3. procedure   4. goals   5. Encourage

Part Two

Task 4

1. no spill cup   2. non-slip bowl   3. utensil hand clip   4. modified utensil

A non-tip cup is the cup that has strong silicone suction on the bottom so that it can prevent the bottle from tipping over by sudden force and accidental hit.

A non-slip bowl is the bowl that has strong silicone suction on the bottom so that it can prevent the bowls from sliding on table.

An utensil hand clip is used to position an eating utensil at a right angle to the palm.

A modified utensil is the utensil that has been modified to assist with difficulties such as reduced grip, tremor or lack of muscle control, use of one hand only, restricted movement and weakness in the arms and shoulders.

Task 5

		1. It doesn't matter. / Never mind.
		2. Don't worry.
√		3. I can really understand that you…
		4. You will recover soon.
√		5. I could see that was hard work for you, but you did a good job.
		6. Don't be nervous. Your doctor is expert for this disease.
√		7. You did a good job. / You did really well.
		8. Please come back to see the doctor for a check-up in two weeks.

Task 6

(N=nurse; A=Anita, patient)

Sample:

N: Hello Anita, here is your lunch.

A: I don't feel like eating.

N: Do you feel sick or uncomfortable?

A: No…I don't feel sick, but I hate to sit here for the whole day. It seems I can't do anything after the stroke. I can even hardly feed myself… I just don't have appetite at all.

N: I can really understand that you don't feel hungry. But your body needs the nutrition so that you can regain your strength and energy. I've got some tools to help you. Maybe you can try and eat on your own.

A: OK…I will try and eat a little bit.

N: These are non-slip bowl and non spill cup.

A: Em… They are good.

N: There are some modified utensils for you, too.

A: What for?

N: These spoons are easier for you to hold.

A: Right, well. I'll try them out.

(Patient eats some of her meal.)

N: You did really well. Did you finish your meal? Or you would like to have some other food?

A: I have done with the meal.

N: May I take these utensils away?

(Patient nods.)

N: I could see that was hard work for you, but you did a good job. You have eaten half of the meal on your own!

A: Thank you.

Part Three

Task 7

1. flexion   2. adduction   3. extension   4. rotation

Task 8

1. √   2. √   3. √   4. √   5. √

7. WNL with no pain   8. WNL with some pain

9. limited to 120°   10. not able to do

Task 9

(N=nurse; P=patient)

N: Hi, Hugo. Are you ready for today's exercise session?

P: I'm a little tired…I feel hopeless. I can hardly play basketball, right? I feel useless.

N: It's common after the shock of such a big car accident. Long stay in bed may make you lose confidence. But you are really doing such a good job of recovering.

P: You think so?

N: Absolutely! You have done very well considering the extent of your injuries. I have noticed that you have fought to recover in such a determined way.

P: Thank you… What's our goal today?

N: Shall we start from ankle? Your goal is three sets of rotations and ten sets of pumps.

P: OK.

N: First move your ankle in a circular motion… good… repeat 5 times in each direction… and one more set. Now push your foot up and down slowly for 10 times… Let's count it together… eight, nine, ten! That's very good. How do you feel?

P: I'm fine.

N: Now for the knee bends exercise. Please keep your heel on the bed and bend the knee… hold it for 3 seconds… then straighten it again…You're doing very well. Try it again. Our goal is 3 sets of 10 on each leg…Good job!

More Practice

(N=nurse; P=patient)

N: OK, Mr. Carter. It's important to do these exercises every day for your recovering.

P: It seems useless…I still can't lift my baby boy…

N: It's not unusual after the fracture. A prolonged hospital stay makes you lose your confidence. But you are making progress.

P: Do you reckon that?

N: Definitely! Your shoulder flexion and extension are getting much better. You might not feel it useful yourself at this moment, but I think it is anything but useless. I have seen how you interact with your little boy. You are gifted in communicating with children. He looks so happy to be with you.

P: Thank you…What are we going to do today?

N: Let's start from the right shoulder. Our goal is 10 sets of shoulder flexion and extension. Is that OK?

P: I'll try.

N: Good. Please move your arms from your side to straight above your head…very good. Then move it back to stick out behind you… Is that your limit?

P: I think so…

N: That has been improving already. I think we could stop here and repeat it 10 times… That's it. Now for 10 sets of abduction and adduction. Do you need some rest?

P: I'm OK. Thanks.

N: Are you ready? Tell me if it hurts, OK?

P: OK.

N: Please place your right hand on top of your head… then move back… Fabulous… Then repeat it… Let's count together… eight, nine, ten! You are on target!

Unit 15

Communication Focus

1. Because you can give the listener an equal chance to speak their mind and respond to what you have said.

2. When I am speaking, I frequently pause for short periods to allow my listener a chance to interject if they need to. When others are speaking, I'll try not to interrupt them, wait until they have finished or at least paused for a few seconds before responding. For some unconfident and weak patients, I will give them plenty of communicative space to express themselves.

Part One

Task 1

1. f   2. d   3. g   4. e   5. a   6. b   7. h   8. c

Examples:

(SA=student A; SB=student B.)

SA: Something is used to help people to walk.

SB: It's a walking stick or a walking frame.

SA: Something is used to help people to slide from the wheelchair onto the toilet.

SB: It's a raised toilet seat.

SA: Something is used to help people to hold on when they take a bath.

SB: It's a grab bar.

SA: Something is used to stop people from slipping in the bathroom.

SB: It's a non-slip mat.

SA: Something is used to help people to take a bath easier.

SB: It's a shower chair.

…

Task 2

ADLs Assessment			
Patient Name: Amy		**Ward: 1**	
Toileting	Independent ☑	Needs assistance ☐	Dependent ☐
Dressing	Independent ☐	Needs assistance ☑	Dependent ☐
Bathing/showering	Independent ☑	Needs assistance ☐	Dependent ☐
Eating	Independent ☐	Needs assistance ☑	Dependent ☐
Ambulation *	Independent ☑	Needs assistance ☐	Dependent ☐
Transferring **	Independent ☐	Needs assistance ☐	Dependent ☑

(**Note**: * getting around on foot   **getting around by vehicle)

Task 3

1. DOD   2. AD   3. DOA   4. DD   5. HOD

Reporting sample:

The patient is called Linda Gilbert, and she is 80 years old. She was admitted because of the left-sided weakness, swallowing and speech difficulties on 7th November 2018. First, she was diagnosed as stroke. The patient was admitted and placed on aspirin, nutritive brain cell and intravenous fluid to ensure the cerebral perfusion, nasal feeding and limb exercise by the attending physician Dr. John Hockings. After two weeks, the patient improved, showing gradual resolution of left-sided weakness, swallowing and speech difficulties. The patient will be discharged in a stable condition. Dr. Hockings prescribed some medications for her. Her follow-up appointment with Dr. Hockings has been made on 21 December at Out-patient Department.

Part Two

Task 4

1. The staff nurse has already sent your prescription to the pharmacy.

2. Let me check about your follow-up appointment with the doctor.

3. Have regular meals and keep a diet of vegetables and fruits.

4. Which exercise should I take?

5. Your follow-up appointment has been made on 10:00 a.m. Wednesday.

6. Continue your low-salt diet after your discharge.

7. Take a tablespoonful three times a day at mealtimes.

8. What are aerobic exercise?

About exercise	About diet	About medication	About follow-up appointments
4 8	3 6	1 7	2 5

Task 5

Dialogue	Patients/care givers' worries			Nurse's advice about mobility aids
	bathing	toileting	dressing	
1		√		raised toilet seat
2	√			grab bars, non-slip mat
3	√		√	shower chair

[Examples]

(N=nurse; P=patient)

1.

N: So, do you think you are going to manage at home?

P: Well, nurse, I am nervous about bathing in the bathroom.

N: Well, it's a good idea to install a grab bar in order for you to hold during bathing.

P: Thank you very much. I will have a try.

2.

N: Is there anything you are worried about?

P: I have a problem to go to the toilet.

N: If you can't go to the toilet yourself, a raised toilet seat will be able to help you.

P: Really? Sounds good.

3.

N: So, do you think you are going to manage at home?

P: I just don't know how I can take my sister to the park while she can't walk.

N: Why don't you buy a wheelchair so you can take her around?

P: That's a good idea! Where can I buy it?

N: You can buy it in our hospital or at any pharmacy.

Task 6

Sample:

(N=nurse; S=Susan, patient)

N: Good Morning, Susan. How are you feeling today?

S: Fine, thanks. I feel great today.

N: Congratulations! Here is a discharge form for you.

S: That's good news! You see I'm really looking forward to going back to work.

N: Don't be in a hurry.

S: How long do you think it will be before I can return to my work?

N: I can assure you that you'll fully recover in three to five weeks.

S: Is there anything I should follow?

N: You'd better have a good rest for one week.

S: You mean I should stay in bed for the whole week?

N: You should go outdoors more and do some exercise.

S: What kind of food should I have, special nourishment?

N: Have regular meals first. Keep a diet of vegetables and fruits. Keep off alcohol. If possible, give up smoking, at least for a time.

S: Should I take some medicines?

N: Yes, your doctor has written a prescription for you. You have to take them every day.

S: When will these tablets be finished?

N: In a week.

S: How should they be taken?

N: Take one tablet of this medicine three times a day before meals. And that one, two tablets once daily in the morning.

S: I see. Thank you.

N: Remember to come to the Out-patient Department for a consultation; your follow-up appointment with Dr. Milton is in a week.

S: All right.

N: You can pack your things and settle the account today.

S: All right, but I must inform my husband first.

N: I have called him for you. He is coming in half an hour.

S: I feel really grateful to you. Many thanks.

N: You are welcome. We wish you an early recovery. Goodbye.

Part Three

Task 7

Saying who you are	Sally speaking.
	It's Tina calling.
Saying why you are calling	I'd like to make a referral.
	I'd like to refer an 80-year-old lady to you for some District Nursing Services.
Asking someone to do something	Could you please spell that for me?
	Could you hold for a minute?
Inquiring about something	Do you want me to give you her daughter's number?
	Does she need her meals delivered to her at home?

Task 8

1. Gilbert   2. Andrea   3. 01254556723   4. Hockings   5. bathing; mobility

6. soft   7. No   8. Yes   9. 12th June   10. walking frame; shower chair

Task 9

Sample:

(M= Milly, District Nurse; S= Sandy, hospital registered nurse)

M: District Nursing Service. Milly Frank speaking.

S: Hello, it's Sandy here from the Alexandra Hospital. I've got an 80-year-old lady I'd like to refer to you for some District Nursing Services. Can I give you the details now?

M: Could you hold on for a minute? I'll get a referral form. OK, I'm ready, er, it was Sandy, wasn't it?

S: That's right. Sandy Clarke from the Alexandra Hospital.

M: Thanks, Sandy. What's the patient's name, please?

S: I've got a Linda Gilbert for you.

M: OK. Could you please spell that for me?

S: Sure. It's L-I-N-D-A, the surname's spelled G-I-L-B-E-R-T.

M: Got it. Linda Gilbert.

S: Her address is 15 Summer Lane, Exeter. It's a bungalow. The spare key's with her next of kin.

M: OK, do you have Linda's home phone number, please?

S: Yes, I've got it here. It's o one two five four, five five six, seven two three.

M: Yes, thanks. O one two five four, five five six, seven two three. Is that correct?

S: Yes, that's right. Do you want me to give you her daughter's number, too?

M: Yes, please.

S: Her daughter's name is Andrea. She is also her next of kin. Her phone number is o one four five six, six seven nine, nine nine eight.

M: Got it. Thanks.

S: Linda's GP is Dr. John Hockings. I'll spell that for you. It's H-O-C-K-I-N-G-S.

M: OK.

S: Linda had a stroke three weeks ago. She's got moderate left-sided weakness and still has some difficulty in swallowing. She needs quite a lot of help with her ADLs, especially bathing and mobility. She's quite unsteady on her feet and uses a walking frame.

M: What will I have to order?

S: She might need a shower chair. But it'd be better to wait until after she has a home assessment done before any aid are ordered. The home assessment has been booked for 12th June.

M: That's Monday, 12th June, right?

S: Yes, that's it. Linda's house will need some adaptions.

M: OK. How's she managed with her diet?

S: She's been managing a soft diet for a few days.

M: Mm, soft diet. Does she need her meals delivered to her at home?

S: No. Her daughters are very supportive. Well, I think I've given you all the information you need. Her discharge summary will be sent to you in the next day or so. Is there anything else you need to know?

M: No. I think I've got everything. Thanks.

S: No problem and thanks for your help.

More Practice

Sample:

(K= Kathy, charge nurse; W= Wendy, daughter of the patient)

K: So, you are Wendy, Eric's daughter? I'm Kathy, Eric's Charge Nurse.

W: Hello, Kathy. I'm informed that my father will be discharged in two days. So I'm here to know more about his current state and the care we should have at home.

K: Oh, we've just had a weekly team meeting about what we've been doing for him to finalize his discharge plan and his expected date of discharge has been put down as Friday, 10th June. That's the day after tomorrow.

W: OK, I see. Can you explain once again about the effect of a stroke and how he has been doing here?

K: No problem. Your father had a left CVA which is affecting his right side. Right, let's look at left CVA first. Ischemia causes death of tissue on the left side of the brain. This causes damage to the body functions on the right side of the body. In the case of a mild left CVA, it causes right-sided weakness. More serious damage in a left CVA causes right-sided paralysis. When your father was admitted, he had got right-sided weakness and it was well over the initial three hours from the onset of the stroke.

W: Yes, his body is quite weak on that side.

K: Our physiotherapist has been helping him with all the physio exercises. He has been trying really hard and has shown gradual resolution of right-sided weakness. But he still needs a lot of help with his ADLs.

W: I see.

K: The weakness affects the muscles around the mouth as well, and this is why swallowing's difficult. The other consequence of having weak muscles around the mouth is difficulty in articulating words, so his speech is affected.

W: Dad's certainly having trouble with pronunciation; he just can't get the words out properly.

K: Yes, the speech and language therapist has also been doing some exercises with him. Fortunately, your father is able to communicate, but he does have difficulty expressing himself. That's why he says the wrong words for the thought he's trying to express.

W: It's really frustrating him. We don't know what to do. Sometimes he just starts crying.

K: Mm, emotional lability is very common. It usually shows up as crying at inappropriate times. Oh, it's very distressing, I know.

W: Oh, OK. Thanks for explaining that. We'll try to be more patient with him. By the way, what should we prepare at home?

K: Your home assessment has been booked for tomorrow. Your house needs some adaptions. After that, you can order some mobility aids, such as a walking frame, a shower chair, etc. A non-slip mat is necessary in the shower.

W: OK. How's he managed with his diet?

K: He's been managing a soft diet. I'm afraid he couldn't prepare meals at least for this period of time. You'd better prepare for him in advance; he or his neighbor can heat them up when you are at work.

W: Thank you for your consideration.

K: Now, do we have your contact details on file?

W: Yes, I gave the nurse my phone number yesterday.

K: OK. Thanks. You can discuss your concerns with me any time you want.

W: Thanks. I appreciate your help.